BASAL CELL CARCINOMA

Edited by **Vishal Madan**

Basal Cell Carcinoma
Edited by Vishal Madan

Published by InTech
Janeza Trdine 9, 51000 Rijeka, Croatia

Publishing Process Manager Molly Kaliman

Technical Editor Teodora Smiljanic

Cover Designer InTech Design Team

Additional hard copies can be obtained from orders@intechopen.com

Basal Cell Carcinoma, Edited by Vishal Madan
p. cm.
ISBN 978-953-51-0309-7

For EU product safety concerns:
IN TECH d.o.o., Prolaz Marije Krucifikse Kozulić 3, 51000 Rijeka, Croatia,
info@intechopen.com or visit our website at intechopen.com.

Meet the editor

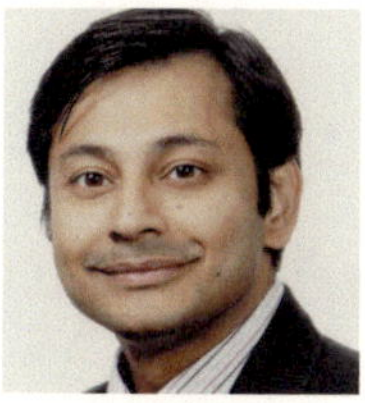

Dr Vishal Madan, MBBS (Hons), MD, MRCP is a Consultant dermatologist, Laser and Dermatological surgeon at the Salford Royal NHS Foundation Trust and Central Manchester Foundation Trust, Manchester, UK. He qualified in Dermatology in India and moved to the UK in 2002. After completing the prestigious Addenbrooke's Cambridge medical rotation, he undertook his specialist training in Dermatology in Manchester. As he has a special interest in procedural dermatology he has completed two fellowships- one in Laser Dermatology at the Salford Royal NHS Foundation trust and another fellowship in Mohs micrographic (Skin cancer) and reconstructive skin surgery at the Welsh Institute of Dermatology, University Hospital of Wales, Cardiff. Dr Madan has published in excess of 95 articles, authored 4 book chapters and edited a book on specialty examination in Dermatology and another on skin cancer. He has been an invited reviewer for 11 international journals and has 50 scientific presentations. Dr Madan runs a successful laser course at the Salford Royal NHS Trust.

Contents

Preface

'Basal Cell Carcinoma' provides an insight into the recent developments and on going research into molecular biology and pathogenesis of basal cell carcinomas. This book also includes a chapter on metastatic basal cell carcinoma, an underreported clinical entity and sheds light on a custom made mold brachytherapy technique for certain basal cell carcinoma subtypes. A detailed account of the genomics of basal cell carcinoma compliments other chapters focusing on the pathogenic mechanisms. It is hoped that this book will offer the readers a greater understanding of the role of cytokines and chemokines and unfold the molecular pathways leading to development of basal cell carcinomas. Understanding of such mechanisms is central to development of targeted therapy which is of much interest to the clinicians and it is hoped that this book will help to facilitate further research into this field.

Dr Vishal Madan MD, MRCP
Consultant Dermatologist, Laser and Dermatological Surgeon
Salford Royal NHS Foundation Trust and Manchester Royal Infirmary,
Stott Lane
Salford, Manchester
M6 8HD
UK

1

Custom Made Mold Brachytherapy

Bahadir Ersu
Hacettepe University Department of Prosthodontics, Ankara
Turkey

1. Introduction

Radiotherapy (RT) can be effective for primary BCC, recurrent BCC or as adjuvant for incompletely excised BCC in patients where further surgery is neither possible nor appropriate. Radiotherapy is a mixture of superficial, electron beam, and brachytherapy for curved surfaces. Treatment in fractions over several visits may produce better cosmetic outcomes than a single fraction treatment.[1] Radiotherapy is contraindicated in radiotherapy recurrent BCC, genetic syndromes predisposing to skin cancer and connective tissue disease. Significant side effects are radionecrosis, atrophy, and telangiectasia. Skin cancers can arise from radiotherapy field scars and should be avoided in younger age groups.

Brachytherapy has been widely used for the treatment of head and neck cancers. Mold therapy is excellent for the treatment of superficial carcinomas because it allows the planning of an adequate dose distribution before treatment and provides highly reproducible irradiation.[2,3] However, therapists and members of the nursing staff can be exposed to radiation if remote afterloading units are not used. Although the combination of mold and remote afterloading units has been used in the head and neck region, including the oral cavity,[4-6] its use as a method of radical radiotherapy has been extremely limited because of the low flexibility of the connection catheters. Recently developed units with 192-Ir microsources have more flexible catheters and molds that are better suited to uneven regions such as the oral cavity. The first case of superficial carcinoma of the nasal vestibule that was successfully treated by a technique combining a mold and a remote afterloading unit with a 192-Ir microsource was reported in 1992.[7] However, no well-controlled case of treatment of an oral carcinoma through use of this combined technique has yet been reported, although trials of interstitial use are now in progress.[8-11] Details on construction of molds used in this type of therapy have been described in the literature.[12] Because of the favorable reports concerning the combined technique, we planned to use it for primary oral carcinomas as a part of radical radiotherapy.

Basal cell carcinoma (BCC) is an epithelial tumor of the skin.[13] It arises from the basal cells of the surface epidermis and can exhibit various clinical manifestations. It predominantly occurs on exposed areas of the skin. Actinic radiation is considered a major etiologic factor. It appears to be directly proportional to the amount of exposure of the skin to sunlight and is inversely proportional to the degree of skin pigmentation. Chronic arsenic exposure and genetic factors may also play a role in the development of BCCs. BCCs are highly variable and several different clinical types are recognized.[13,14]

Various methods have been used for treatment of BCC. These techniques have included electrocoagulation followed by curettage, electrosurgery, chemosurgery, chemotherapy, and radiation therapy.[13,14] Radiation therapy can be delivered either by external beam radiation or by brachytherapy. Brachytherapy is usually applied in the form of interstitial therapy, which involves the implantation of radioactive sources into the tissues or the application of radioactive molds to the skin surface.[15] Mold brachytherapy is usually delivered in specially constructed carriers. Surface radiation carriers primarily indicated for the treatment of superficial lesions. They are helpful where external radiation can be used as a boost dose.[13] Such carriers can vary in design from the simple to complex, according to treatment needs.[14] The radiation carrier should be easy to fabricate and be readily usable by the radiation oncologist. Carriers that will be worn for extended periods must be carefully constructed to provide maximal patient comfort and to ensure at the same time correct dose delivery to the treatment area and reproducibility of the treatment at repeated sessions. An irreversible hydrocolloid is used for making impression. The carrier can be constructed from autopolymerizing acrylic resin rather than heat-curing acrylic resin. Cerrobend alloy is chosen for shielding purposes.[16]

2. Mold production procedure

It consisted of a mold of polymethyl methacrylate (PMMA) of 5 mm thickness, built over a plaster mold obtained as an individual impression of the region of the face to be treated. The construction of this PMMA mold was very similar to the construction of dental prostheses. First, an impression of the region of the patient to be treated was obtained with condensation silicones of putty texture (Optosil, Bayer), carefully adapted to the surface of the skin with gentle pressure. Over this impression a plaster model was obtained, with the same surface characteristics as the patient's face. Over this plaster model, the contours of the tumor were carefully drawn, requiring generally the presence of the patient. Over this plaster model, successive thin layers of acrylic material with catalyzer were deposited, until a minimum thickness of 5 mm was obtained, taking care to avoid sharp surfaces. This first layer of PMMA had to act as a bolus material and as a first support for the brachytherapy catheters. On it, the appropriate number of plastic tubes, covering the area to be treated, were fixed with an instant contact glue. Usually 3 to 7 parallel and equidistant tubes were placed, following the contour of the zone to treat, parallel to the skin's surface and avoiding sharp turns. The distance between the catheters ranged between 5 to 10 mm. The next step was to check that the radioactive source ran without interruption along the entire length of the catheters, by connecting the tubes to the microselectron and running the check cable. In case of curvatures of a diameter smaller than that required to pass the microselectron source through the tube, the plastic tube was replaced and glued in a new position, checking again the pass of the source through the catheters. Only when the source passed through all channels without any problem, was the custom mold completed by adding the necessary quantity of PMMA acrylic material and catalyzer to cover all the catheters and to give solidity to the mold. To harden the assembly, it was heated to 70°C for 5 minutes with a hair dryer, taking care to avoid deformations of the guide tubes. In the sides of the applicator were built some, usually two, buttonholes in which an elastic tape was fixed to maintain the mold in the correct position during the entire treatment time and facilitating the reposition of the assembly for daily treatment. Treatment parameters were calculated by the 3D treatment planning software (Plato, Nucletron Int. BV). Each source dwell position was weighted individually to ensure the best isodose distribution. Geometrical optimization in volume and distance was done. Isodoses at skin surface and at 5-mm depth were plotted and the dose to 5 easily identifiable dose points calculated. The treatment parameters were chosen, with the best fit of isodoses to the target volume. Before treatment, a test run without the patient was done: the mold was attached to the plaster model with 5 thermoluminescent dosimeters (TLD) placed in the dose points and guide tubes connected to the microselectron. The results of the TLD were read and compared with the calculated values. A verification autoradiograph of the applicator was obtained modifying the prescribed dose to 50 cGy to the film but maintaining the same weight to each dwell time. In the cases of tumors close to the eye, a lead sheet 5 mm thick was placed in the corresponding zone of the mold in order to reduce the dose to the eye. The procedure of construction, dosimetry, and verification of the custom-made mold required 3 working days, requiring 2 visits of the patient before beginning the treatment, one to take the impression of the face and the second to draw the tumor and treatment volume on the plaster model. The custom-made applicators were used to treat tumors of more than 2 cm diameter, or those of smaller size but seated in a non-flat region or a difficult-to-fix area with the Brock's applicators. In one patient it was necessary to built a second mold at the halfway point of the treatment, due to changes in the surface of the skin resulting from tumor regression.

2.1 Tolerance of custom-made molds

All patients tolerated treatment without difficulties. Patients helped the nurses to fit the custom-made mold in place. Treatment time took 3 to 8 minutes in each session. The custom-made molds were very ease to use, and the patients felt comfortable during treatment. There were no cases of interruption of treatment resulting from break of the applicator or constriction of the plastic tubes preventing the radioactive source from traveling properly to the treatment dwell positions.

2.2 Conclusions

Radiotherapy is a highly effective treatment of skin carcinomas of the face and head. The use of HDR brachytherapy with custom-made external molds permits one to obtain a uniform dose distribution with a sharp gradient in the edges of the applicator. The custom-made molds are easily used and permit a highly accurate daily treatment reproduction. They enable one to obtain excellent local control with minimum treatment-related sequelae or late complications. Given the excellent results, HDR brachytherapy with external custom-made molds is a reasonable alternative to other radiation therapy techniques for the treatment of skin carcinomas of the head and face.

3. Clinical reports

3.1 Case report 1: A hinged flange radiation carrier for the scalp

The purpose of this cases was to describe fabrication of a hinged flange radiation carrier for a patient with BCC of the scalp.

A 63-year-old man with the chief complaint of scalp lesions of 15 years duration was examined at the Hacettepe University hospital. These lesions were biopsied and diagnosed as BCC (Fig. 1). Radiation treatment of 4 days duration (details could not be obtained) to the scalp performed 45 years ago was noted in the patient's history. Total scalp excision was suggested as the treatment of choice. However, the patient refused the surgical intervention because of cosmetic problems and was accordingly referred to the department of radiation oncology. The treatment that was selected was a specially constructed mold suitable for remotely controlled after-loading brachytherapy. The patient was referred to the department of prosthodontics for fabrication of the radiation carrier

3.1.1 Procedure

The catheter radiation carrier was fabricated to ensure the fixation of the after-loading catheters in the required orientation to make the treatment reproducible. For fractionated treatment, it was decided to fabricate a catheter carrier mold. The patient's head was shaved, and the border of the shaved area was outlined on the skin with indelible pencil. The patient's head was lubricated with petroleum jelly (Aafes). The moulage impression of his head was made with irreversible hydrocolloid impression material (Blueprint Cremix, Dentsply, DeTrey, England) supported with gypsum (Kristal Alçi Sanayi Ltd., Ankara, Turkey). The surface was outlined with a pencil and boxed with wax. The impression was then poured in dental stone. One layer of baseplate wax (1 mm in thickness) was adapted over the cast. The catheters were placed parallel to each other at spaces of 10 mm (Fig. 2). The spacing was determined by the radiation oncologist and the radiation physicist in accordance with dosimetry for the target volumes to avoid creating cold or hot spot areas in the treatment region. Autopolymerizing methyl methacrylate (Meliodent, Bayer Dental, Bayer UK Limited Bayer House, Newbury, U.K.) was prepared, poured, and spread over the surface. The device was designed to be two pieces from frontal to cervical border. An acrylic resin hinge was fabricated and embedded into the two pieces (Fig. 3, *A* and *B*). This approach was necessary because undercuts over the head prevented placement of the carrier as a single unit. After polymerization and trimming, the device was tried on the patient's head and adjusted (Fig. 4). Remote control after-loading technique was used to provide radiation and to distribute the active sources in the mold. High dose rate (HDR) microselection equipment with Ir-192 source and 1.77 ´ 1011 Bq activity was used. A total dose of 4050 cGy at 0.5 cm skin depth was given over a period of 3 weeks.

3.1.2 Discussion

Radiation prostheses have assisted the delivery of radiotherapy for carcinomas. These prostheses are used to protect or displace vital structures from the radiation field, locate diseased tissues in a repeatable position during radiation treatment, position the radiation beam, carry radioactive material or dosimetric devices to the tumor site, recontour tissues to simplify the therapy, or shield tissues from radiation. Radiotherapy has been used in the management of the head and neck region for many years. It has been shown to be effective in the treatment of superficial lesions. [15,16] Superficial lesions usually have a higher cure rate with radiation than do deeply infiltrating lesions. Radiation treatment of BCC is reported to be 96.4% with radiation therapy.[17] Small BCCs that occur in essential cosmetic area can be successfully treated with a short treatment course[14] (Fig. 5). Surgery is indicated, especially when the lesions have arisen in damaged skin or have invaded cartilage.[18] Modern brachytherapy is delivered by remote controlled after-loading systems where the radioactive sources are delivered to the prepositioned treatment catheters HDR remote control after-loading brachytherapy is used in the treatment of patients with curative intent.[19] There are several advantages in using HDR remotely controlled after-loading systems. Radiation exposure of treating and nursing staff is virtually eliminated. Patient immobilization time is short; therefore complications that result from prolonged bed rest, such as pulmonary emboli and patient discomfort, is decreased. Treatment planning and dosimetry are more exact. Radioactive sources can be accurately positioned to a specific region. The sources have been arranged for loading according to the results of calculations by the radiation physicist to determine dose distribution. This ensures delivery of the calculated degree of radiation. If a change in dosage is required, it can be adjusted accordingly. Treatment can be performed on an outpatient basis, reducing healthcare cost. The use of external carrier fixation devices allows more constant and reproducible geometry for source positioning. Surface radiation carriers are being used more frequently with high dose remote after-loading devices.[19]

3.1.3 Conclusions

A hinged flange cranial radiation carrier was fabricated for a patient with basal cell carcinoma of the scalp. This method allowed for accurate and repeatable positioning of the carrier to facilitate radiation therapy. The use of the after-loading principles of brachytherapy allowed for the delivery of an accurate dose of radiation while minimizing radiation exposure to the radiation oncologist and nursing staff. The patient is in complete remission 15 months after treatment.

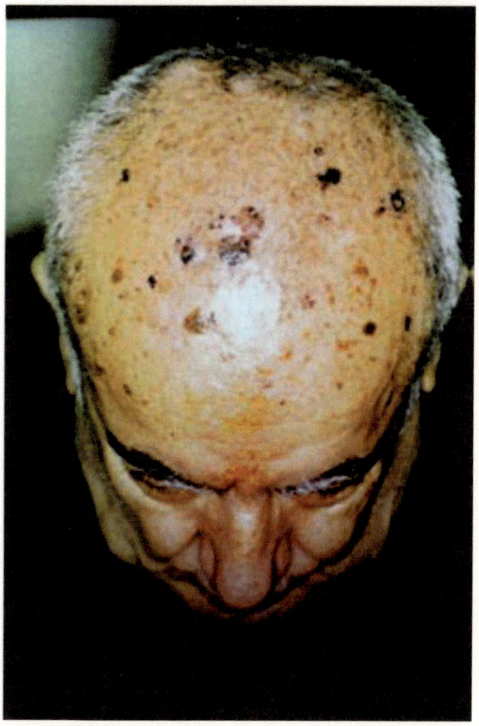

Fig. 1. View of patient with lesions on scalp.

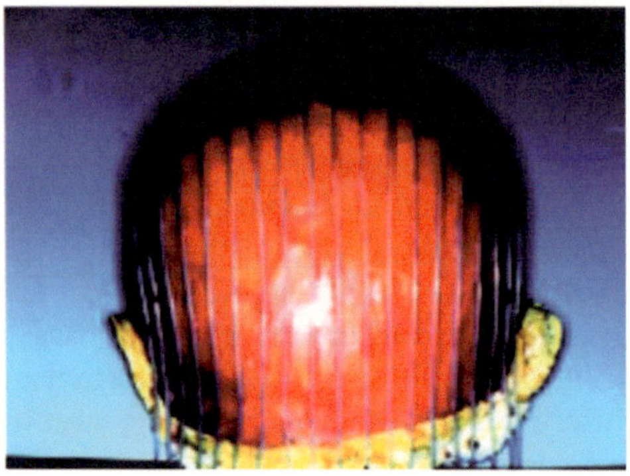

Fig. 2. Catheters were embedded within wax plates and placed parallel to each other at intervals 10 mm on cast.

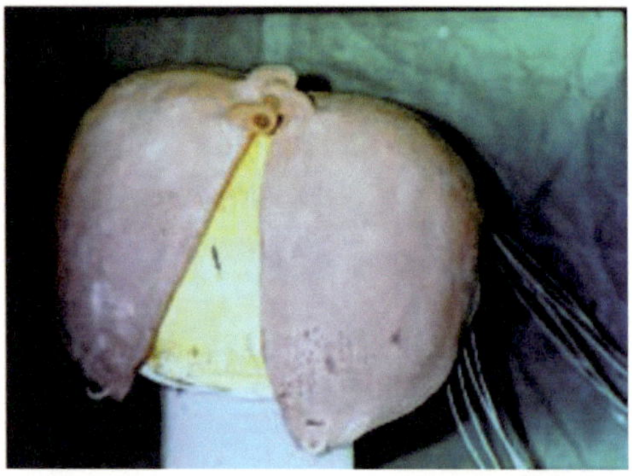

A

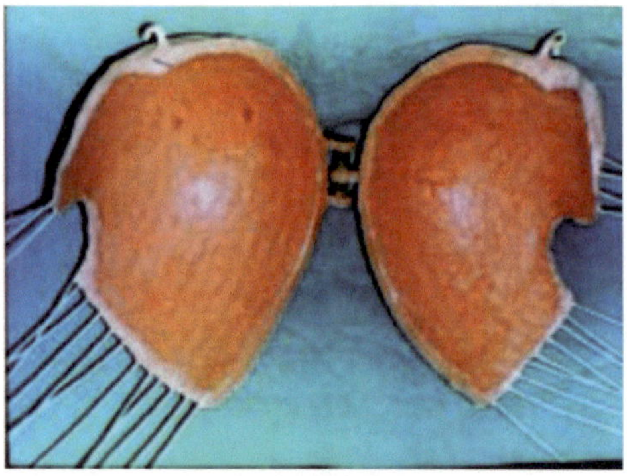

B

Fig. 3. **A,** Outer view of carrier on cast. **B,** Inner view of carrier.

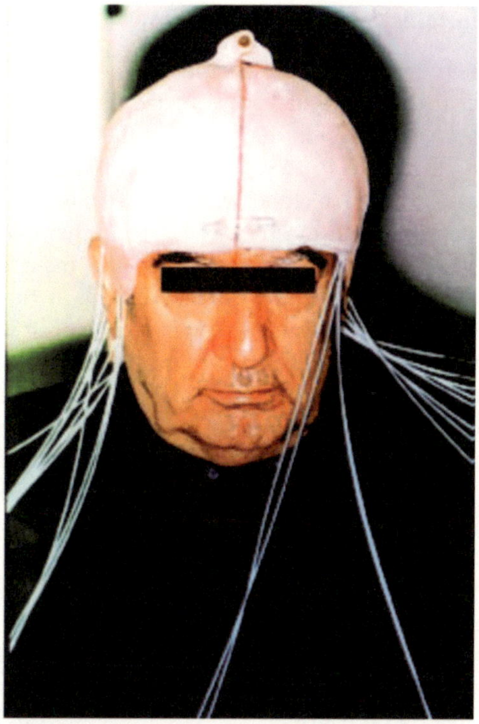

Fig. 4. Radiation carrier is placed and fixed on patient's head.

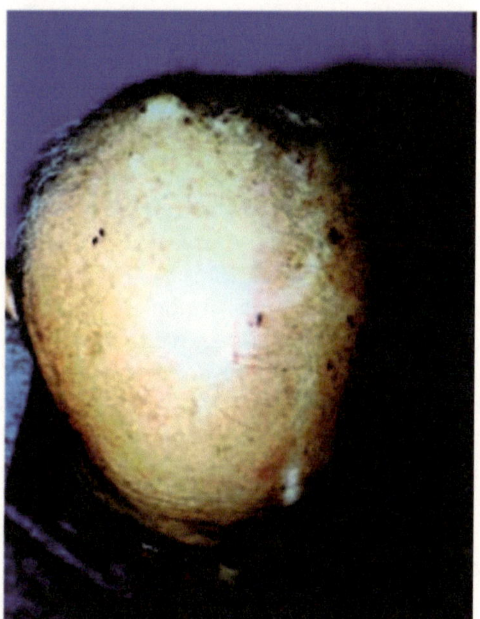

Fig. 5. View of patient's scalp 15 months after radiation treatment.

3.2 Case report 2: Periauricular mold brachytherapy

A 42-year-old male was referred to the Otorhinolaryngology Department of Hacettepe University with the clinical diagnosis of recurrent BCCA of the right pinna (Fig. 6). The patient was treated in 1992 for a lesion in the periauricular area that was totally excised and pathologically diagnosed as BCCA. In 1995, a recurrent BCCA lesion infiltrating into the parotid gland was excised; and in October 1995, a retroauricular recurrent BCCA was excised and the patient treated with electron beam radiotherapy at the dose of 5000 Gy using fraction size of 250 Gy in 1996. In October 1996, a recurrent BCCA in the fronto-parietal area was excised; and in 2000, a recurrent BCCA in the remaining right auricle infiltrating to the mastoid process was excised. A recurrent tumor was then diagnosed in the mastoid cavity in September 2001 and a final attempt at excision of the tumor was made with known microscopic residual disease. It was then decided to treat the patient with brachytherapy. The patient was informed about possible severe side effects of the treatment, and the patient was referred to the Department of Prosthodontics for fabrication of a radiation carrier. The patient was reclined in dental chair; the head positioned allowing the patient to rest in a relaxed position with easy application of impression material to the lesion area. The neighboring area with hair was isolated with petroleum jelly, and the orifice of the outer auricular canal was filled with moist gauze. The external border of the area that was intended to be included in impression was outlined with utility wax (Moldwax; Sankay Ltd., Izmir, Turkey). An irreversible hydrocolloid impression material (Kromopan; Lascod Sp.H., Firenze, Italy) was mixed and poured over the target area and slightly pushed and directed to the desired areas with a brush. Then, a simple wrought wire metal mesh was applied over the impression material for eliminating possible distortions that may occur during the removal of the impression and subsequent setting of the cast. The impression was poured with a Type III dental stone (Amberok, Ankara, Turkey). A 0.5-mm thick layer of pink modeling wax plate (Multiwax; B.D.P Industry, Ankara, Turkey) was heated slightly and adapted onto the model to act as a spacer preventing the direct contact of catheters to the tissues, extending through the borders of the target area (Fig. 7). To avoid developing hot or cold spots, the spaces between the plastic carrier tubes (Nucletron; Veenendaal, Netherlands) and the space between tubes and tissues were standardized by the use of wax sheets of uniform thickness. The catheters were placed parallel to each other with 8 mm distance. As the surface of the target tissue was not perfectly smooth, the adaptation of catheters to the superficial contours of these areas was impossible; two catheters were superimposed in these areas where needed (Fig. 8). The mold was prepared with clear autopolymerizing acrylic resin (Akribel; Atlas- Enta, Izmir, Turkey) overextending 2 mm from the treatment area. The wax spacer was removed, and this area was filled with a soft-lining material (Visco-Gel; Dentsply De Trey, Konstanz, Germany) to provide an excellent adaptation of the radiation mold to the target area (Figs. 9 and 10). A remote-controlled high-dose-rate (HDR) after-loading unit (microselectron; Nucletron) was used for the treatment. Q4The CTV defined as 5-mm tissue starting from the surface Q5 of the mold and therefore encompassing microscopically residual tumor volume. Dose calculations were performed using Plato brachytherapy treatment planning system (Nucletron). The dose was specified at the reference dose-rate curve encompassing the CTV. A total radiation dose prescribed to the reference isodose was 2500 cGy in 10 fractions in an overall treatment time of 5 days. The patient did well during and after the treatment. The patient was lost to followup, after followed in complete remission for 2 years.

3.2.1 Discussion

Radiotherapy has been used in the adjunctive management of the head and neck region for many years. It has been shown to be effective in the treatment of superficial lesions [20,21]. Superficial lesions usually have a higher cure rate with radiation than do deeply infiltrating lesions [20]. Successful radiation treatment of BCCA is reported to be 96.4% with radiation therapy [28]. Small BCCAs that ocur in critical cosmetic areas may be successfully treated with a short treatment course [21]. Radiation delivery devices are important for delivery of radiotherapy and are used to protect or displace vital structures from the radiation field, locate diseased tissues in a repeatable position during succeeding radiation treatment sequences, position the radiation beam, carry radioactive material or dosimetric devices to the tumor site, recontour tissues to simplify the therapy, or shield tissues from radiation [20,21]. However, the technique of implanting radioactive materials into target tissues may have potential disadvantages. The major concern is the potential for nonuniformity of the dose delivered throughout the implanted volume. This can occur if the radioactive sources are spaced too closely together (thereby producing a hot spot) or too far apart (leading to a cold spot). Therefore, brachytherapy (and particularly interstitial implantation therapy) requires the radiotherapist to have adequate technical and conceptual skills to achieve good radiation dose distribution [29]. Some clinicians have stated that most patients who have had radiation treatment for malignancies will, in time, develop new cancers in the irradiated area. Experienced radiotherapists who carefully followed their patients for many years find this to be an extremely rare possibility and irradiation should never be withheld from the patient for this reason. The best local control results for patients with previously irradiated recurrent head and neck cancers were reported to be with brachytherapy [30]. The reason for better local control was argued in the literature and reported that tumors with good prognostic factors (smaller tumors and oral cavity locations) were suitable for treatment with brachytherapy. Moreover, higher radiation dose could be delivered by brachytherapy [30]. Our patient was previously received high-dose external beam radiation, tumor and we decided to deliver reirradiation with brachytherapy. Q7 We delivered 25 Gy in 5 days, divided in 10 fractions. Most authors used similar fractionation; however, most used higher doses. Narayana et al. [31] also delivered HDR brachytherapy, a total dose of 34 Gy in 10 fraction, twice daily, and reported 2-year local control rate of 71% for recurrent squamous cell carcinoma of the head and neck. Martinez-Monge et al. [32] also delivered HDR brachytherapy for previously irradiated recurrent head and neck carcinomas, the authors used 40 Gy in 10 fractions and achieved 4-year local control rate of 85.6%. We have only one case and unfortunately we could not report long-term followup. Because of basal carcinoma histopathology and prior external beam radiotherapy, we think that 25 Gy would be enough to achieve local control. There are many advantages of using HDR remotely controlled after-loading radiation delivery systems that cannot be overlooked. This method takes advantage of the rapid decrease in dose with distance from a radiation source (inverse square law). The intensity of radiation is inversely proportional to the square of the distance from the source. Thus, a high radiation dose can be given to the tumor while sparing the surrounding normal tissues. Patient immobilization time is short; therefore, complications that result from prolonged bed rest, such as pulmonary emboli and patient discomfort, are decreased. Treatment planning and dosimetry are more exact. Radioactive sources can be accurately positioned to a specific region. The sources have been arranged for loading according to the results of calculations by the radiation physicist to determine dose distribution. This ensures accurate delivery of the calculated magnitude of radiation. If a change in dosage is required, it can be adjusted accordingly. The use of external carrier fixation devices allows more constant and reproducible geometry for source positioning. Surface radiation carriers are being used more frequently with highdose remote after-loading devices [23].

3.2.2 Conclusion

This method allowed accurate and repeatable positioning of the radiation carrier to facilitate therapy. Carriers that will be worn for extended periods must be carefully constructed to provide maximal patient comfort and to ensure, at the same time, correct dose delivery to the treatment area and reproducibility of the treatment at repeated sessions. Mold brachytherapy is an option for reirradiation of recurrent head and neck tumors in selected group of patients.

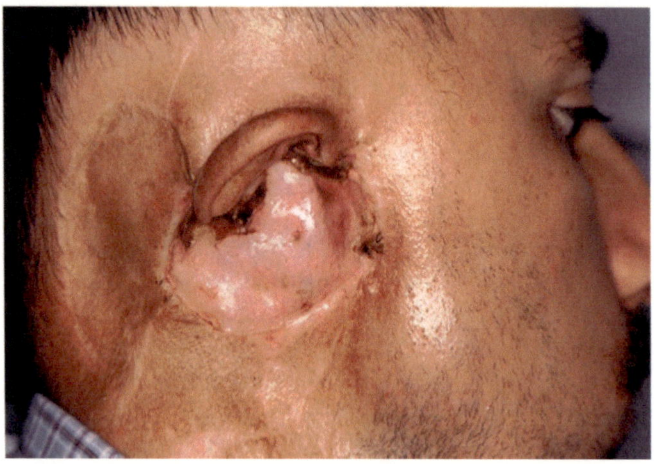

Fig. 6. Patient with recurrent basal cell carcinomas of right periauricular area.

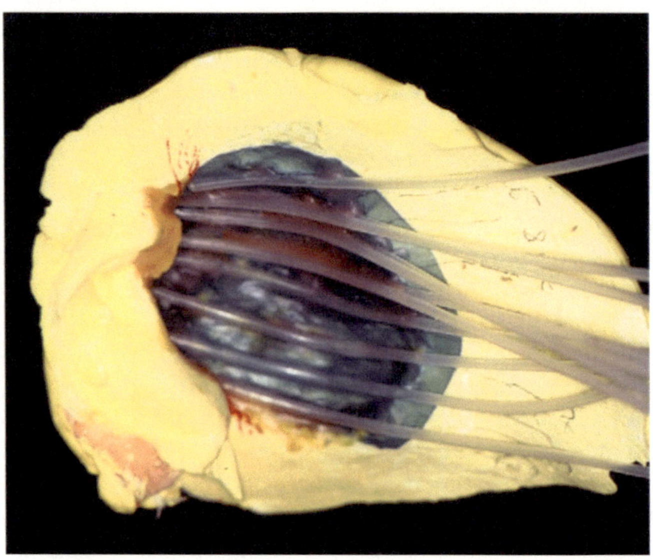

Fig. 7. Wax spacer and placement of catheters.

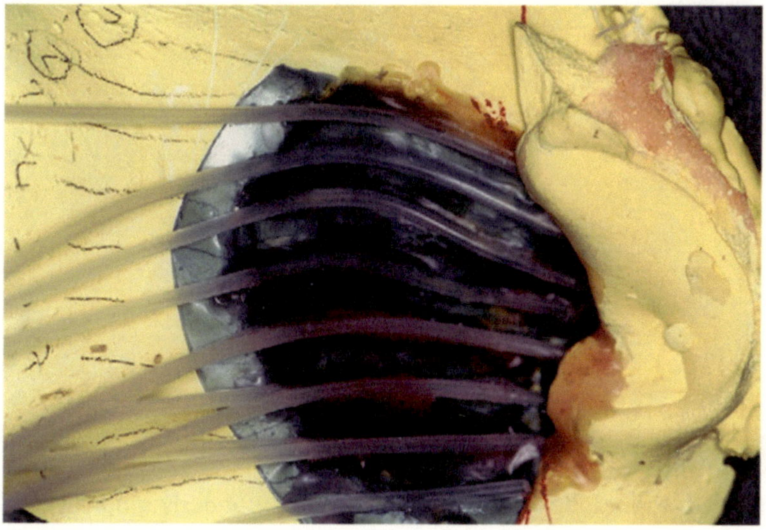

Fig. 8. Two catheters were superimposed in irregular areas.

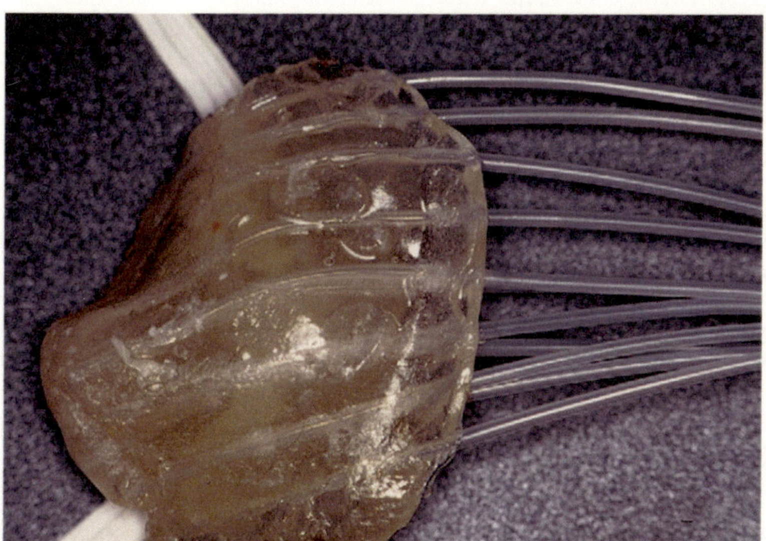

Fig. 9. Wax spacer removed and replaced with soft-lining material.

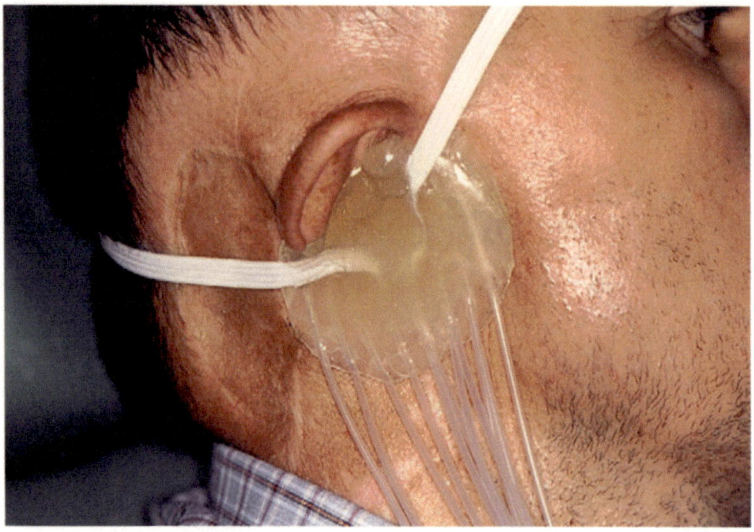

Fig. 10. Adaptation of brachytherapy appliance to target tissues.

3.3 Case report 3: High dose rate mold brachytherapy of early gingival carcinoma

The purpose of this clinical report is to present the use of mold brachytherapy in the management in gingival cancer.

Gingival carcinomas are rare, constituting less than 2% of all head and neck tumors.[33] Surgery with intraoral resection of the tumor or wide excision with the underlying bony structures is the most preferred treatment approach.[33] Radiation therapy is used as an adjunct to surgery and is the primary treatment modality in inoperable patients.[33,34] Radiotherapy can be applied either through external beam or by brachytherapy. However, mold brachytherapy is rarely used in the management of the head and neck tumors, it is a promising method with encouraging results.[35] It has the advantages of low acute radiation morbidity and shortened treatment period compared with the external beam technique.

3.3.1 Patient 1

A 70-year-old edentulous woman was seen by her dentist with the complaint of ill-fitting dentures, which had been experienced for 2 months. A tumoral lesion that measured 25 × 15 mm was detected in the left maxillary gingiva. A biopsy was performed on the lesion (Fig. 11); histopathologic examination of the specimen was consistent with well-differentiated squamous cell carcinoma. She denied use of alcohol or tobacco, and it was learned that she had been wearing dentures for more than 30 years. The computerized tomography (CT) of the primary tumor and neck region showed no abnormality. The patient was staged as T2NOMO cancer of the maxillary gingiva and referred for primary radiation therapy. High dose rate (HDR) mold brachytherapy was applied, considering the size, site, stage and differentiation of the tumor, and age of the patient (Fig. 12).

Brachytherapy was well tolerated without any acute side effects. Grade IV mucositis was observed immediately after the treatment and healed completely in 1 month. Complete regression of the tumor was observed 1 month after the treatment (Fig. 13). The patient is alive and disease-free 36 months after the treatment.

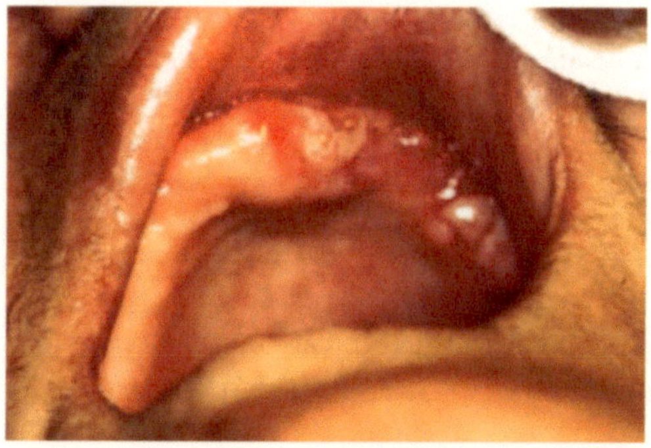

Fig. 11. Tumoral lesion at left side of maxillary gingiva before brachytherapy.

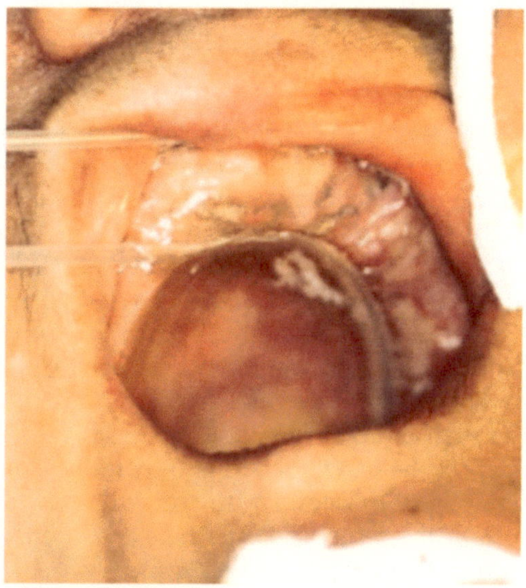

Fig. 12. Application of mold brachytherapy.

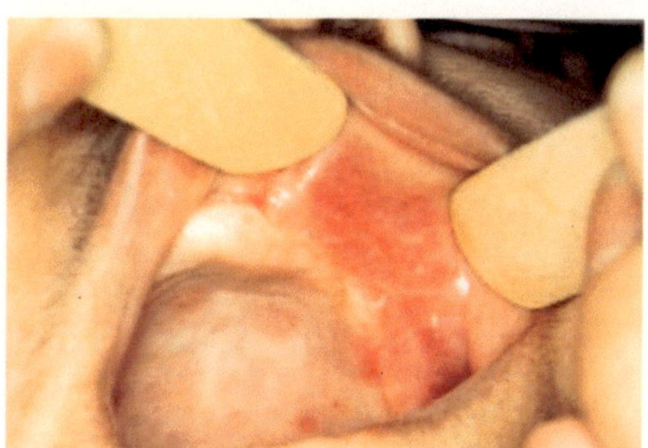

Fig. 13. Lesion from Figure 2, 1 month after brachytherapy, shows complete response.

3.3.2 Patient 2

A 84-year-old edentulous woman with a 6-week history of an ill-fitting denture was admitted to the hospital at Hacettepe University. Physical examination revealed a tumoral mass that measured 30 × 15 mm on the maxillary left gingiva and leukoplakia on the neighboring mucosa. A biopsy specimen of the lesion disclosed moderately differentiated squamous cell carcinoma. There was no pathologic lymph node on physical examination and CT scan. The patient had a history of using dentures for the last 26 years and no history of alcohol or tobacco consumption. The patient was staged as T2NOMO carcinoma of the maxillary gingiva and referred to radiation therapy. Brachytherapy by customized dental mold was planned. No acute side effects were observed. However, grade III mucositis developed after the completion of treatment. Although complete resolution of tumor was achieved, the patient experienced dyspnea due to pleural effusion at the sixth month of follow-up. Her condition gradually deteriorated and she died of intercurrent disease with pleural metastases 6 months after the brachytherapy.

3.3.3 Procedures

3.3.3.1 Dental mold

Irreversible hydrocolloid impressions of the maxillae were made for both patients and custom trays were fabricated onto the obtained cast. Final impressions were made with a medium viscosity additional cure silicone material (Coltene/Whaledent Inc, Mahwah, N.J.) and were poured in type III dental stone (Amberok, Ankara, Turkey). After trimming the post-dam area, 2 layers of modeling wax were heated and adapted onto the cast to obtain a uniform thickness denture base. The cast was then flasked, the elimination of wax was accomplished with hot water, and heat-cured acrylic resin (Meliodent Bayer, Newbury, Berkshire, U. K.) was used to process the stent. After deflasking and trimming away excess material, the tubes that would transport the radioactive source to the target site were placed into the resin base preserving approximately 10 mm distance between each other. Two plastic tubes of 6F diameter for the first patient (Fig. 14) and 4 tubes of the same types were used for the second patient (Fig. 15). Grooves were formed on the base to allow the tubes to closely contact the mucosa at the target site. The tubes were ending at the border of the target site and secured with clear autocuring acrylic resin.

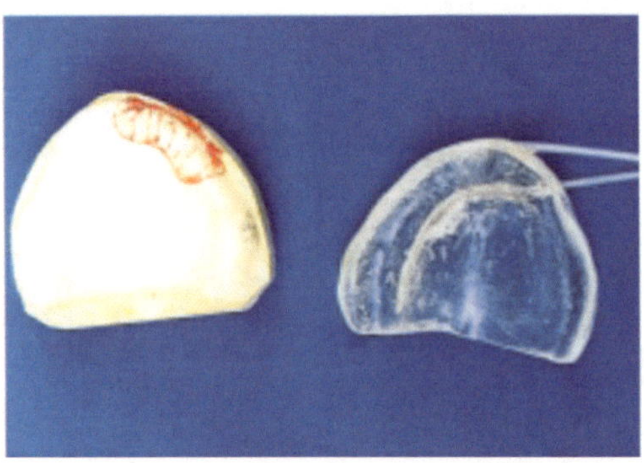

Fig. 14. Impression of maxillary gingiva and tumor using irreversible hydrocolloid paste (right) and acrylic resin dental mold with 2 6F plastic catheters incorporated within it, parallel to gingiva (left).

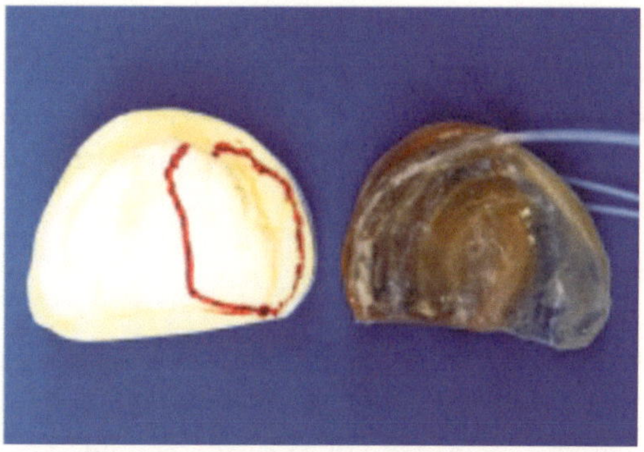

Fig. 15. Impression of maxillary gingiva and tumor of second patient (right) and acrylic resin dental mold with 4 6F plastic catheters incorporated (left).

3.3.3.2 Brachytherapy

Position of the dummy sources within the tubes were verified by simulation. Dosimetric calculations were performed by using the Plato Nucletron planning system (module BPS, Nucletron B.V., Veenendaal, The Netherlands). Irradiation was delivered by an Ir-192 HDR micro Selectron Afterloading unit. A total of 40 Gy was administered in 4 Gy fractions twice daily in 10 fractions and overall treatment time of 5 days for both patients. Special intraoral shielding lead blocks were used to shield buccal mucosa and tongue. Biologically equivalent doses for both patients were calculated to be 56 Gy10 for the tumor and 120 Gy2 for the late reacting tissues. Reference dose rate was 264.6 cGy/min and total air kerma was 0.06 cGy at 1 m for the first patient and 162.7 cGy/min and 0.12 cGy at 1 m for the second patient. The active length of both sources were 2.5 cm and the dimensions of the specified reference dose volume was 3.5 × 2.5 × 1.5 cm for the first patient. Active length of the sources were 4.25 cm for 1 source and 4.75 cm for the remaining 2 sources of the second patient. The specified reference dose volume was 4 × 4.5 × 3.5 cm for the second patient.

3.3.4 Discussion

Gingival carcinomas are rare tumors and optimal treatment modality is not settled yet. Early lesions are mostly treated with surgery, the role of definitive radiotherapy in these cases is unclear. External beam radiotherapy is generally used postoperatively or rarely as a primary treatment in advanced lesions.[33,34] Mold brachytherapy experience in oral cavity carcinomas is mostly with low dose rate brachytherapy.[35-37] There are few reports in the literature on the use of HDR mold brachytherapy combined with or without external beam therapy and the optimal time; dose and fractionation for HDR brachytherapy has not yet been determined.[38-40] In 1 of these reports, an early carcinoma of the nasal vestibule was treated with HDR mold brachytherapy and treatment parameters of this patient were similar to our patients.7 After an extensive literature review, only 1 report was found on the use of dental molds with HDR remote brachytherapy.[41] Eliminating the morbidity of surgery, preserving the function of major salivary glands, being an outpatient treatment procedure, and allowing simple repeated noninvasive treatments are the advantages of HDR mold brachytherapy. Inadequate previous experience is the major disadvantage of this technique. Although the follow-up period is relatively short, these patients seemed to indicate that HDR mold brachytherapy alone may be used in the management of small volume cancers of the gingiva with satisfactory local control. It was presumed that brachytherapy may be used as a boost method after external beam radiation for larger lesions. Because there is not enough experience and data in oral cavity cancers of HDR brachytherapy, more patients should be treated to determine the optimal dose and fractionation.

3.3.5 Summary

Two elderly edentulous patients with the diagnosis of early stage cancer of the upper gingiva were treated by customized dental mold brachytherapy. Locoregional tumor control was achieved in both patients. One patient is alive without any evidence of disease 36 months after treatment, the other patient died of distant metastasis shortly after brachytherapy. Brachytherapy, being easy to apply with short treatment time and good acute tolerance, is a good choice and effective modality for the management of early stage gingival cancer, particularly in elderly patients.

4. References

[1] Telfer NR, Colver GB, Morton CA. Guidelines for the management of basal cell carcinoma. British Journal of Dermatology. 2008;159(1):35–48.
[2] Rustgi SN, Cumberlin RL. An afterloading 192-Ir surface mold. Med Dosim 1993;18:39-42.
[3] Takeda M, Shibuya H, Inoue T. The efficacy of gold-198 grain mold therapy for mucosal carcimonas of the oral cavity. Acta Oncol 1996;35:463-7.
[4] Joslin CAF, Eng C, Liversage WE, Ramsey NW. High dose-rate treatment molds by afterloading techniques. Br J Radiol 1969;42:108-11.
[5] Miyata Y, Inoue T, Nishiyama K, Ikeda H, Ozeki S, Hayami A, et al. Remote afterloading high dose rate intracavitary radiotherapy for head and neck cancer. Nippon Acta Radiologica 1979;39:53-9.
[6] Bauer M, Schulz-Wendtland R, Fritz P, von Fournier D. Brachytherapy of tumor recurrences in the region of the pharynx and oral cavity by means of a remote-controlled afterloading technique. Br J Radiol 1987;60:477-80.
[7] Pop LA, Kaanders JH, Heinerman EC. High dose rate intracavitary brachytherapy of early and superficial carcinoma of the nasal vestibule as an alternative to low dose rate interstitial radiation therapy. Radiother Oncol 1993;27:69-72.
[8] Itami J. Clinical application of high dose rate interstitial radiation therapy. Nippon Acta Radiologica 1989;49:929-40.
[9] Teshima T, Inoue T, Ikeda H, Murayama S, Furukawa S, Shimzutani K. Phase I/II study of high-dose rate interstitial radiotherapy for head and neck cancer. Strahlenther Onkol 1992; 168:617-21.
[10] Teshima T. High-dose rate brachytherapy for head and neck cancer. Japanese Journal of Clinical Radiology 1994;39:1127-34.
[11] Inoue T, Inoue T, Teshima T, Murayama S, Shimizutani K, Fuchihata H, et al. Phase III trial of high and low dose rate interstitial radiotherapy for early oral tongue cancer. Int J Radiat Oncol Biol Phys 1996;36:1201-4.
[13] Beumer J, Curtis TA, Firtell DN. Maxillofacial rehabilitation. St Louis: CV Mosby; 1979. p. 23-40.

[14] Chalian V, Drane JB, Standish SM. Maxillofacial prosthetics. Baltimore: Williams & Wilkins; 1971. p. 251-6.
[15] Hope-Stone HF, editor. Radiotherapy in modern clinical practice. 1st ed. London: Granada Publishing Ltd; 1976. p. 13-4.
[16] Beumer J, Curtis TA, Firtell DN. Maxillofacial rehabilitation. St Louis: CV Mosby; 1979. p. 36.
[17] Brash DE. Cancer of the skin. In: DeVita VT, Hellmano S, Rosenberg SA, editors. Cancer—principles and practice of oncology. 5th ed. Philadelphia: Lippincott-Raven; 1997. p. 1879-933.
[18] Rafla S, Rotman M. Introduction to radiotherapy. St Louis: CV Mosby; 1974. p. 158-9.
[19] Perez CA, Garcia DM, Grigsby PW, Williamson J. Clinical applications of brachytherapy. In: Perez CA, Brady LW, editors. Principles and practice of oncology. 2nd ed. Philadelphia: JB Lippincott; 1992. p. 300-67.
[20] Chalian VA, Drane JB, Standish SM. Maxillofacial prosthetics. Baltimore: The William and Wilkins Company; 1972. p. 181-183.
[21] Vandeweyer E, Thill MP, Deraemaecker R. Basal cell carcinoma of the external auditory canal. Acta Chir Belg 2002;102:137-140.
[22] Nyrop M, Grontved A. Cancer of the external auditory canal. Arch Otolaryngol Head Neck Surg 2002;128:834-837.
[23] Tanigushi H. Radiotherapy prostheses. J Med Dent Sci 2000;47: 12-26.
[24] Ray J, Worley GA, Schofield JB, et al. Rapidly invading sebaceous carcinoma of the external auditory canal. J Laryngol Otol 1999; 113:873.
[25] Sheiner AB, Ager PJ. Delivering surface irradiation to persistent unresectable squamous cell carcinomas: A prosthodontic solution. J Prosthet Dent 1978;39:551-553.
[26] Ozyar E, Gurdalli S. Mold brachytherapy can be an optional technique for total scalp irradiation. Int J Radiat Oncol Biol Phys 2002;54:1286.
[27] Cengiz M, Ozyar E, Ersu B, et al. High-dose-rate mold brachytherapy of early gingival carcinoma: A clinical report. J Prosthet Dent 1999;82:512-514.
[28] Ahmad I, Das Gupta AR. Epidemiology of basal cell carcinoma and squamous cell carcinoma of the pinna. J Laryngol Otol 2001;115: 85-86.
[29] Beumer J, Curtis TA, Marunick MT. Maxillofacial rehabilitation: prosthodontic and surgical considerations. St. Louis: Ishiyaku Euroamerica Inc.; 1996. 49-50.
[30] Kasperts N, Slotman B, Leemans CR, et al. A review on re-irradiation for recurrent and second primary head and neck cancer. Oral Oncol 2005;41:225-243.
[31] Narayana A, Cohen GN, Zaider M, et al. High-dose-rate interstitial brachytherapy in recurrent and previously irradiated head and neck cancers-Preliminary results. Brachytherapy 2006;6:157-163.
[32] Martinez-Monge R, Alcade J, Concejo C, et al. Perioperative highdose-rate brachytherapy (PHDRB) in previously irradiated head and neck cancer: Initial results of a Phase I/II reirradiation study. Brachytherapy 2006;5:32-40.
[33] Million RR, Cassisi NJ, Mancuso M. Oral cavity. In: Million RR, Cassisi NJ, editors. Management of head and neck cancer: a multidisciplinary approach. 2nd ed. Philadelphia: JB Lippincott; 1994. p. 321-400.
[34] Soo KC, Spiro RH, King W, Harvey W, Strong EW. Squamous carcinoma of the gingiva. Am J Surg 1988;156:281-5.

[35] Mold RF. Head and neck brachytherapy before and after loading. Selectron Brachytherapy J Suppl 1992;3:88-9.

[36] Parsai E, Ayyangar K, Bowman D, Huber B, Dobelbower RR. 3-D reconstruction of Ir-192 implant dosimetry for irradiating gingival carcinoma on the mandibular alveolar ridge. Oral Surg Oral Med Oral Pathol Oral Radiol Endod 1995;79:787-92.

[37] Shibuya H, Takeda M, Matsumoto S, Hoshina M, Suzuki S, Tagaki M. The efficacy of radiation therapy for a malignant melanoma in the mucosa of the upper jaw: an analytic study. Int J Radiat Oncol Biol Phys 1992;25:35-9.

[38] Pop LA, Kaanders JH, Heinerman EC. High dose rate intracavitary brachytherapy of early and superficial carcinoma of the nasal vestibule as an alternative to low dose rate interstitial radiation therapy. Radiother Oncol 1993;27:69-72.

[39] Fietkau R. Brachytherapy for head and neck tumors. Activity Selectron Brachytherapy J 1993;27:69-72.

[40] Otti M, Stuckischweiger G, Danninger R, Poier E, Pakisch B, Hackl A. HDR brachytherapy for hard palate carcinoma. Activity Selectron Brachytherapy J 1992;Suppl 3:26-8.

[41] Jolly DE, Nag S. Technique for construction of dental molds for high dose rate remote brachytherapy. Spec Care Dent 1992;12:219-24.

2

Molecularbiology of Basal Cell Carcinoma

Eva-Maria Fabricius, Bodo Hoffmeister and Jan-Dirk Raguse
Clinic for Oral and Maxillofacial Surgery, Campus Virchow Hospital
Charité – Universitätsmedizin Berlin
Germany

1. Introduction

Basal cell carcinoma is the most frequently occurring skin tumor. Most cases are not life threatening. Only a very small proportion of BCCs metastasize. A high tendency to recurrence makes characterizing BCCs and tumor margin areas obligatory. It will assist in better understanding their pathogenesis and in more effective treatment through prevention of recurrence and second primary disease. In addition to histopathological assessment, the spread of the primary tumor according to TNM classification is crucial for estimating the further development of the disease.

1.1 Molecular alterations involved in the emergence and development of basal cell carcinomas (BCC)

While it has not been fully clarified which primary cell gives rise to basal cell carcinomas it is supposed that BCCs arise from interfollicular basal cells, keratinous cells of hair follicles or sebaceous glands (1 to 6). Chemically induced BCCs were produced in the pilosebaceous structures of rats (3, 7). Solar ultraviolet radiation (UVR), in particular ultraviolet B (UVB, waveband 280-315 nm), is a major and significant factor (8 to 23) in many of the carcinogenic steps leading to basal cell carcinomas. Additional risk factors are predisposing syndromes and genetic predisposition (3, 11 to 14, 16, 19, 24 to 41), such as skin-type (13, 42, 43), viral infections, above all human papilloma viruses (HPV) and / or immunosuppression (3, 13, 17, 20, 35, 39, 41, 44 to 46). The influence of UVB is evident from the fact that BCC incidence is lowest in Finland (47, 48) and highest in Australia (13, 47 to 51). Incidence increases with advancing age through the accumulation of UV-radiation (52, 53). UVB exposure and chronic oxidative stress (54) effect direct DNA damage, mutations and chromosome aberrations in the skin (41, 55 to 57), all of which are found in basal cell carcinomas. They are comparable with squamous cell carcinomas (58) insofar as field cancerization can be shown in the environment of the BCC (59 to 63). The BCC can be characterized by certain markers such as proof of p53. Figure 1 illustrates UVB damage with regard to the mutation and inactivation of tumor suppressor gene p53 as well as activation of telomerase during cancerization, particularly in basal cell carcinomas (64).

The inactivation of tumor suppressor activity is a universal step in the development of human cancers (65, 66). With inactivation p53 looses its function as the "guardian of the genome" (66) thanks to which it normally controls, among other things, the normal cell cycle, arresting irregularly growing cells via G1 / G2 transition of the cell cycle and compelling them to programmed suicide, apoptosis (67 to 76). bcl-2 can block and control p53-dependent apoptosis and loss of bcl-2 stimulates apoptosis (67 to 71, 73, 77, 78). While wild-type p53 suppresses cell growth, p53 mutations reduce DNA repair, for example after UVB radiation, and stop apoptosis. That can explain the increased incidence of skin tumors such as basal cell carcinoma through UVB radiation (13, 79 to 82).

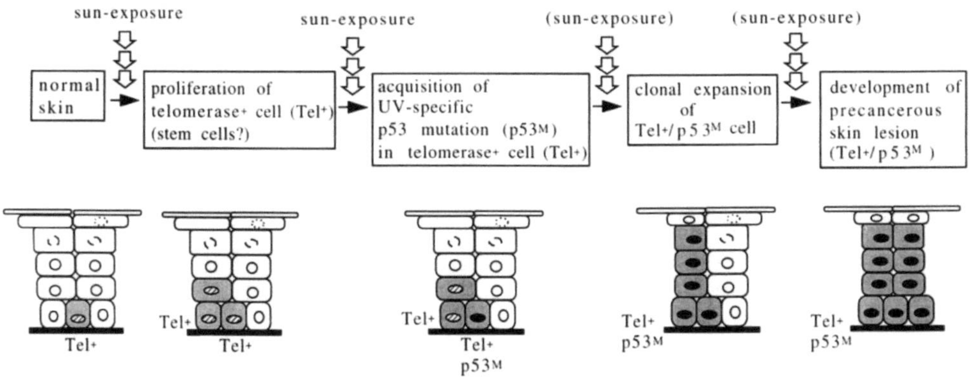

Fig. 1. Carcinogenesis of basal cell carcinomas. Concept for the course of molecular changes in the cancerogenesis of basal cell carcinomas: adapted and reprinted by permission of the American Association for Cancer Research: Ueda et al. (64) (Tel+ = telomerase activation).

1.2 Molecular markers for differentiation of BCC and SCC of the skin

Basal cell carcinomas and squamous cell carcinomas of the skin are differentiated by means of histopathological staining, mostly with hemalaun-eosin staining. This can lead to difficulty, as seen for instance in cytology. Vega-Memije et al. (83) introduced Papanicolaou staining to successfully distinguish between the two carcinoma types, and this was also used by Christensen et al. (84) along with May-Grünwald-Giemsa staining for the cytological differentiation of BCCs and actinic keratosis. Tellechea et al. (85) used immunohistochemical anti-Ber-EP4 monoclonal antibody. The total of 22 BCCs showed positive reactions, while in 21 SCCs the reaction was negative, proving this monoclonal antibody suitable for differentiating between the two nonmelanomatous skin-tumors. It was confirmed by Beer et al. (86) who verified expression of Ber-EP4 in all of 39 BCCs and in none of 23 SCCs tested. Swanson et al. (87) were able to distinguish BCCs both from SCCs of the skin and from trichoepitheliomas (TE) with proven expression of Ber-EP4 (also of bcl-2 and CD34): The reaction of Ber-EP4 was positive in all of 44 BCCs, in 81% (29/36) of TEs and in none of 22 SCCs. According to the same procedure, Tope et al. (88) differentiated between BCC, actinic keratosis (AK) and SCCs: All of 5 superficial BCCs were Ber-EP4 positive, while all of 10 AKs and of 8 SCCs were negative. To differentiate between BCCs and SCCs the Ber-EP4 marker is the most suited. Swanson et al. (87) differentiated with CD34 BCCs, SCCs and TEs: CD34 was positive in 16% (7/43) of BCCs, in 25% (5/20) of SCCs and in 8% (3/36) of TEs. Likewise, Yada et al. (89) and Aiad and Hanout (90) were able to discriminate BCC from SCC immunohistochemically with CD10. In the study by Yada et al. (89) BCCs expressed CD10 1+ to 2+ in 86% (44/51) and in all 9 SCCs CD10 was negative. According to

Aiad and Hanout (90) CD10 expression was significantly higher in BCCs than in SCCs: 10/21 (48%) and 0/16 SCC (p=0.002).

Guttinger et al. (91), Seelentag et al. (92), Dietrich et al. (93) and Seiter et al. (94) used immunohistochemical methods with monoclonal anti-CD44s and various anti-CD44 splice variant antibodies to differentiate BCCs and SCCs. Guttinger et al. (91) obtained distinct marking of tumor cells (++) in all SCCs with anti-CD44s, CD44v4, CD44v6 and CD44v9 antibodies. The nodular BCCs showed no expression and the sklerodermiform BCCs (+) a weaker expression. This result was congruent with studies by Seelentag et al. (92). Seelentag et al. observed the expression of CD44s, CD44v3, CD44v4, CD44v6 and CD44v9 in immunohistochemical paraffin sections. They (92) achieved higher or distinctly higher expression of CD44v3, CD44v5, CD44v6 and CD44v9 in SCCs of the skin (n=37) than in BCCs (n=10). In BCCs the expression was low (CD44s, CD44v3) or absent (CD44v4). Higher expression in BCCs was found with the splice variants CD44v5, CD44v6 and CD44v9. In squamous cell carcinomas Seelentag et al. (92) found CD44v3, CD44v5, CD44v6 and CD44v9 expression comparable with that in keratoacanthomas (n=12). CD44s and CD44v4 expression was lower in SCCs than in keratoacanthomas. This contradicted the findings by Dietrich et al., (93) who demonstrated CD44v4, CD44v5 and CD44v6 both in BCCs (n=7) and in SCCs (n=6). Indeed, using immunohistochemical methods Dietrich et al (93) demonstrated expression of CD44v7/8 and CD44v10 in all BCCs but in none of the SCCs tested. Forming groups according to the estimated percentage of staining cells, Seiter et al. (94) assessed expression of CD44s, CD44v5, CD44v6, CD44v7, CD44v7/8 and CD44v10 semiquantitatively. In the BCCs and SCCs they investigated, CD44s was expressed in the same degree, while all splice variants tested showed higher expression in SCCs. Simon et al. (95) checked the suitibility of immunohistochemistry for definite distinction between BCCs and SCCs with splice variants CD44v3, CD44v4, CD44v5, CD44v6, CD44v7/8 or CD44v10. All splice variants stained the tumor center of BCCs, while in SCCs only tumor periphery was marked. 12/17 BCCs (71%) were positive with CD44v3 and 13/17 (77%) with CD44v5. The remaining CD44-splice variants marked all BCCs, and all of 16 SCCs were marked with all CD44-splice variants. In an immunohistochemical study by Son et al. (96), 49% of BCCs and only 35% of SCCs showed CD44v6 marking.

Al-Sader et al. (97) sought to differentiate immunohistochemically the proliferative indices between BCCs and SCCs. The median scores of the mitotic index were 5 for BCCs and 4 for SCCs (p=0.621), but the authors (97) observed that the median scores of Ki-67 were significantly different, amounting to 271 (per 1000 cells) in BCCs and 340 (per 1000 cells) in SCCs (p=0.029). To differentiate BCCs from skin-SCCs, Park et al. (98) used immunohistochemical proof of p53, p63 and survivin. With p53 the authors were unable to differentiate between the two, which were malignant in differing degrees: 90% 2+ to 3+ vs. 100% 2+ to 3+. Proof of p63 made this distinction possible: BCC 90% 2+ to 3+, SCC 40% 2+, as did proof of survivin (BCC 40% 2+, SCC 80% 2+ to 3+). However, Bäckvall et al. (99) succeeded in demonstrating a significant difference between normal skin adjacent to BCC and that adjacent to SCC (p<0.05) with regard to the number of p53 clones. Chang et al. (100) found significantly less Ki-67 in 10 BCCs investigated (mean score value 12±7) than in 8 SCCs (mean score value 47±21), (p<0.05), and detected clearly different expression of p53 (mean score value BCC 50±17 vs. SCC 61±15). Son et al. (96) used immunohistochemical findings of Ki-67 and p53 to differentiate BCCs (n=108) from SCCs (n=94). Ki-67 expression was low in 90% of BCCs and high in 10%, while Ki-67 showed high expression in 27% of SCCs and low expression in 73%. p53 was demonstrated in 15% of BCCs and in 46% of SCCs. Bolshakov et al. (101) succeeded in establishing clear differences between aggressive SCCs / nonaggressive SCCs and also aggressive BCCs / nonaggressive BCCs through mutation frequency of p53 with single-strand conformation polymorphism and sequencing: frequency of p53 mutations amounted to 35% (28/80) of aggressive SCCs vs. 50% (28/56) of nonaggressive SCCs as opposed to 66% (35/50) of aggressive BCCs vs. 38% (37/98) of nonaggressive BCCs. Chang et al. (100) also demonstrated a clear differentiation between BCC and SCC by immunohistochemical bcl-2 detection: All of 10 BCCs displayed positive marking that was absent in all of 8 SCCs. In consonance with this, Delehedde et al. (80) found immunohistochemically distinct bcl-2 expression (+++) in 17 BCCs examined, which was missing in all of 14 SCCs ($p<0.05$). Likewise, Swanson et al. (87) found positive bcl-2 reaction in 91% (41/45) of BCCs and in 18% (4/22) of SCCs. Contrary to these results Al-Sader et al. (97) observed no difference between the median scores of the apoptotic index in BCCs (10.5 apoptotic cells / 1000 cells) and in SCCs (10 apoptotic cells / 1000 cells).

In our studies we introduced proof of telomerase activity to differentiate BCCs from SCCs (102 to 104), cf. 2.4.1: the proportion of BCCs with activation of telomerase amounted to 87% (26/30) and was barely higher than in SCCs of the skin with 75% (9/12). This result is in approximate conformity with synoptic references: activation of telomerase in 87% (177/203) of BCCs examined altogether and in 77% (58/75) of SCCs of the skin (103, 104). However, our studies demonstrated that the score values of immunohistochemical proof with APAAP (105) of the telomerase subunit hTERT cannot be used to differentiate between BCCs (n=24) and SCCs (n=7) of the skin (106, 107): BCC mean score value 9.4±4.9 (Ab 1: anti-hTERT antibody Calbiochem, USA, code 582005) and 9.0±4.0 (Ab 2: anti-hTERT antibody code NCL-hTERT Novocastra, UK, clone 44F12,) vs. SCC mean score value 9.9±2.4 (Ab 1) and 9.1±3.8 (Ab 2), cf. 2.4.2.

2. Molecular markers for basal cell carcinomas and tumor-free margin tissues

Adequate resection of BCCs is of utmost importance in preventing recurrence (108 to 114). Other authors are therefore searching for markers which discriminate between basal cell carcinoma and histopathologically tumor-free margin. In addition to histopathological assessment, assessing the spread of the primary tumor (T1<2cm, T2 ≥2cm) according to the TNM classification (115) is crucial for assessing further development of the disease. The risk of recurrence of each tumor is defined as closely as possible to enable choice and application of the most appropriate clinical procedure (51, 116, 117). Tumor size is important for prognosis of the disease, as is shown by comparison in Kaplan-Meier curves. With all due precaution given the many censored cases, we ascertain that patients with primary T2 tumors relapse much earlier than those with T1 tumors (Log-rank $p=0.003$): after 14±2 months (T2) vs. 65±16 months (T1), Figure 2.

The classification in nonaggressive basal cell carcinomas and aggressive BCCs is predominantly determined by the clinical course of BCCs and by the tendency to recurrence: nonaggressive nodular, micronodular or superficial BCCs and aggressive infiltrative or morphea BCCs (20, 81, 118 to 121). Additional markers will help to characterize and are essential for distinctly determining the spread of BCCs (19).

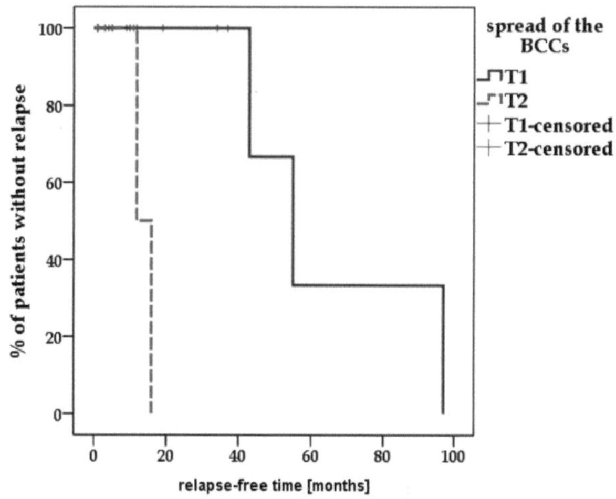

Fig. 2. Up-to-date outcome in patients with BCCs and the spread of the tumor (T1 < 2cm, T2 ≥ 2cm) in Kaplan-Meier curves.

2.1 Different markers classifying nonaggressive and aggressive BCCs

Staibano and colleagues classified between nonaggressive BCC1 without relapse and aggressive BCC2 with local recurrence during metaphylaxis. For this differentiation they introduced various markers. They detected high expression of p53 in 60% of 30 BCC2 tumors and low expression in 10% of BCC1 tumors (122), or in 0/21 BCC1 tumors and in 82% (18/22) of BCC2 tumors, respectively (123). Bolshakov et al. (101) were also able to discriminate clearly between aggressive BCCs and nonaggressive BCCs through determination of p53 mutations by single-strand conformation polymorphism and nucleotide sequencing: the frequency of p53 mutations was 66% (33/55) with aggressive BCCs and only 38% (37/98) with nonaggressive BCCs. In 11 aggressive BCCs Ansarin et al. (121) found significant immunohistochemical nuclear staining of p53 in more than 50% of tumor cells and in 33 nonaggressive BCCs in less than 50% of tumor cells ($p<0.01$).

In BCC1 tumors the AgNOR scores were 6.56±1.98 and in BCC2-tumors 9.48±2.12: De Rosa et al. (119). When Staibano et al. (124) ascertained the apoptotic index, they found a marked difference: BCC1 5.98±2.52% vs. BCC2 39.82±8.32%. BCC1 tumors examined showed a distinct cytoplasmic staining of bcl-2. This marker was missing in all of the 30 BCC2 tumors examined by Staibano et al. (122). In agreement with these investigations Ramdial et al. (81) detected a distinctly higher bcl-2 expression in immunohistochemical assays in nonaggressive BCCs than in aggressive BCCs: 45/50 (90%) nonaggressive BCCs expressed bcl-2 2+ to 4+ and 22/25 (88%) aggressive BCCs maximally 2+. High expression of cyclin D1 was not found in any BCC1 tumors but in all of 30 BCC2 tumors (125). By determining DNA ploidy Staibano et al. (125) were also able to differentiate between BCC1 and BCC2: All BCC2 tumors were aneuploid as against 77% of BCC1 tumors. After immunohistochemical staining for monoclonal antibody against factor VIII (von Willebrand factor), microscopic counts of microvessels revealed a statistically significant difference: mean score value BCC1 25.76±2.21 vs. BCC2 46.76±2.54 (126). Histopathological diagnostics using these markers can be supplementary evidence for the surgeon deciding on the surgical procedure for therapy.

2.2 Examination of BCC spread by means of anti-CD44 antibodies and anti-splice variant antibodies, by anti-E48 and anti-U36 antibodies

Cell adhesion molecules such as CD44 splice variants can be used as selective markers for different tumors and are important both for the diagnosis and prognosis of some tumors (127 to 129). Squamous cell carcinomas with poor differentiation display downregulation of CD44v6 expression in comparison with squamous cell carcinomas with high differentiation. Hyckel et al. (130) planimetered the immunohistochemical reaction of oral SCCs by anti-CD44 monoclonal antibodies and confirmed an inverse relation to carcinoma grading. Our immunohistochemical findings in frozen sections with APAAP (105) in regard to squamous cell carcinomas of the head-and-neck region (131 to 133) are comparable with the downregulation of isoforms containing CD44v6 that Salmi et al. (134) observed with CD44v3 and CD44v6 in SCCs in the head-and-neck area.

Guttinger et al. (91), Baum et al. (135), Seelentag et al. (92), Seiter et al. (94), Simon et al. (95), Kooy et al. (136), Dingemans et al. (137, 138) and Son et al. (96) used immunohistochemical marking on BCCs with CD44v6 and found it better than hemalaun-eosin staining for identifying their local spread. In 20 BCCs, Seelentag et al. (92) found low or no expression of CD44s or CD44v4, contrary to SCCs with low expression of CD44v3. The authors found high expression of CD44v5, CD44v6 and CD44v9 in BCCs, but the expression was lower than in SCCs.

We had previously achieved better results discriminating squamous cell carcinomas of the head and neck from their surroundings with immunohistochemical APAAP (105) in small frozen sections by using adhesion molecules CD44v6 (also its chimera U36) and E48 (131 to 133). This method was now confirmed in BCCs. We accomplished APAAP (105, cf. 131, 132) with a monoclonal antibody against the adhesion molecule CD44v6 (clone VRR-18, Bender, Austria) and with two monoclonal antibodies against adhesion molecules E48 (Centocor B.V., Netherlands) and U36 (Centocor B.V., Netherlands). Antibody E48 has been developed to recognize normal squamous epithelium and squamous cell carcinomas (139). It is well suited for differentiating carcinomas from negative adenocarcinomas and small cell carcinomas (140). Monoclonal anti-U36 antibody is an anti-CD44v6-chimeric (mouse/human) antibody for marking normal human squamous epithelia and squamous cell carcinomas (141 to 143). The quantitative presentation of antigen expression (CD44v6, E48, U36) in frozen sections was evaluated in our study by means of an immunoreactive score (IRS) according to Remmele et al. (144) and Remmele and Stegner (145). Our evaluation was performed three times by an independent examiner. The membrane staining intensities (SI) were divided into 5 levels: negative, 1+ (weak expression) to 5+ (very strong expression). The percentage of positive stained cells (PP) was classified into 4 groups according to percentage of stained cells: 0-<10%=score 1; 10-<50%=score 2; 50-<75%=score 3; 75-100%=score 4. The IRS was calculated by multiplication of SI and PP. To identifying the spread of BCCs in small frozen sections we applied immunohistochemical staining with APAAP (105) to membrane marking of CD44v6, E48 and U36. We found it better than hemalaun-eosin staining.

In our study the immunoreactive scores (IRS) in BCC tumor center vs. tumor-free margin were demonstrated and are illustrated in Figure 3. Only the expression of CD44v6 was significantly higher in tumor center (mean score value 12.5±3.2) than in squamous epithelia in the tumor margin (mean score value 8.4±4.0, p=0.006), and was comparable to the expression of Ki-67 (p<0.001). Microscopic representation with the three monoclonal antibodies, particularly CD44v6, distinguished BCCs clearly from their surroundings: Figure 4.

The ample expression of CD44v6 and U36 (if necessary E48) adhesion molecules might make them useful both for the diagnostics and adjuvant therapy of BCCs. Radionuclide-labeled purified monoclonal antibodies were successfully developed in VU University Medical Center (Amsterdam/Netherlands). They have proven themselves in this capacity for years in the diagnostics (146 to 152) and therapy (142, 147, 153 to 156) of squamous cell carcinomas in the head-neck-region.

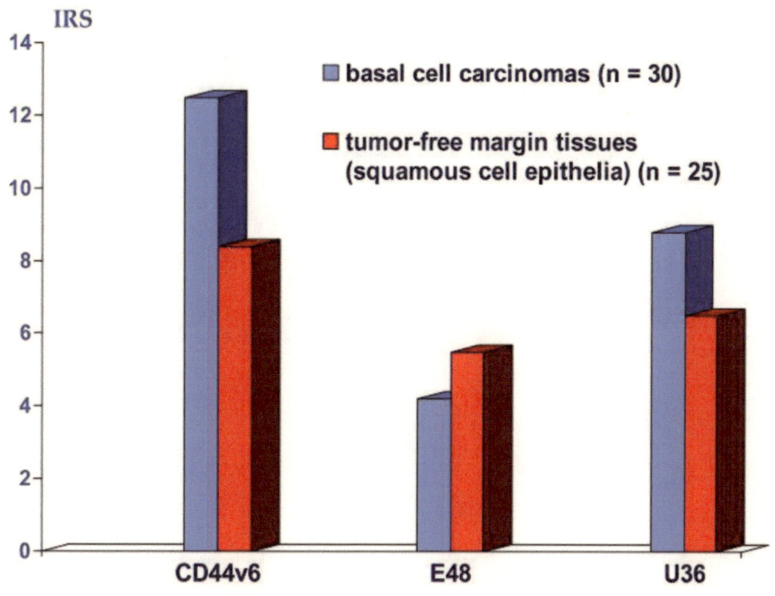

Fig. 3. Immunoreactive scores (IRS, cf. 144, 145) of expression of CD44v6, E48 and U36 in basal cell carcinomas (mean values).

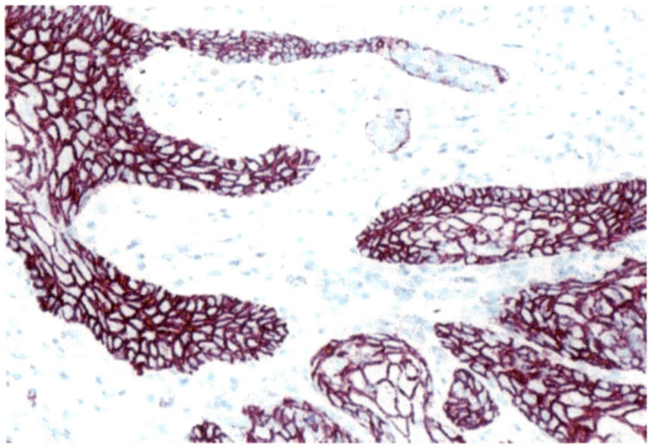

a) CD44v6

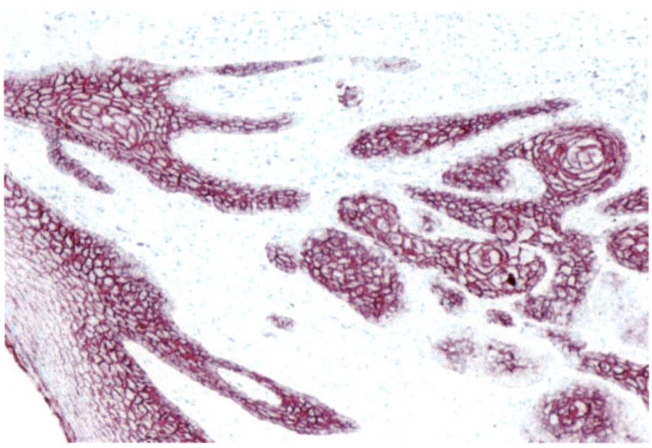

b) E48

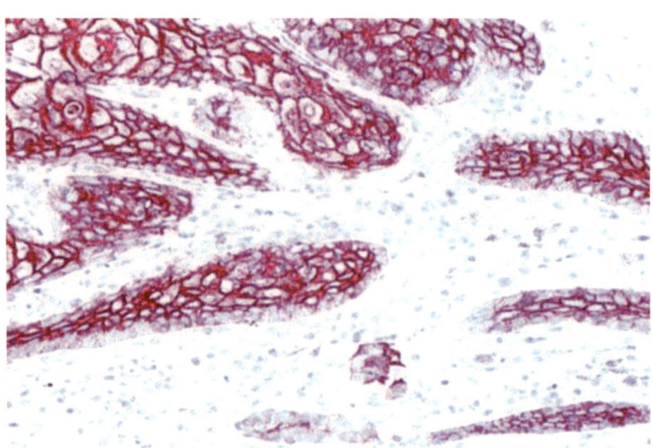

c) U36

Fig. 4. Comparison of expression of CD44v6 (a), E48 (b) and U36 (c) in small frozen sections of BCCs, magnification 200x.

2.3 Markers p53 and Ki-67 in BCCs and BCC-free tumor margin tissue

Molecular alterations can be found during carcinogenesis and tumor growth. As illustrated schematically in Figure 1 (cf. 1.1), the inactivation of tumor suppressor gene p53 is an important step towards carcinogenesis. During inactivation and mutation of p53 mutated p53 protein is formed. Mutated and wildtype p53 protein can be detected immunohistochemically by different or identical antibodies, for instance in tissues with field cancerization after intensive solar irradiation (60, 62) as well as in tumor-free margin surrounding of BCCs (98, 157 to 161). Authors are therefore searching for markers such as p53 which discriminate between basal cell carcinoma and histologically tumor-free margin surrounding the tumor.

2.3.1 Marker p53 in BCCs and BCC-free tumor margin tissues

Urano et al. (157) applied immunohistochemistry using anti-p53 antibody clone Do-7, which recognizes both wildtype p53 protein and mutated p53 protein. The authors found significantly lower p53 expression in tumor margin than in tumor center ($p<0.05$): 7/17 tissues of tumor margin (41%) and 11/17 (65%) of tumor center were p53 positive. Barrett et al. (158) were able to detect p53 in 20/27 (74%) BCCs. They also investigated adjacent actinic keratosis in the tumor margin of 4 tumors and found increased p53 staining. Demirkan et al. (159) detected significantly less p53 in BCC-free tumor margin than in the tumor center: 26% (11/42) p53 positive tumor-free margins vs. 44% (8/18) tumor center tissues ($p=0.034$), the same was found with monoclonal antibody Do-7 (DAKO/Denmark). According to investigations by Rajabi et al. (160), p53 expression in 96/123 BCC tumor tissues (82%) was not significantly higher than in 84/117 tumor-free margin tissues (78%), $p=0.38$. The relatively high p53 expression of the tumor margin could be related to strong sun exposure of uncovered skin with patients in southern latitudes. Bäckvall et al. (99) and Koseoglu et al. (161) were also unable to find a significantly decreased expression of p53 in adjacent tissues surrounding the BCCs. Koseoglu et al. (161) detected p53 clones in 10/43 tumor center tissues (23%) and in 9/21 tumor margin tissues (42%).

In our study we employed an antibody from Oncogene (USA) to ascertain p53 scores in small frozen sections: a monoclonal antibody against mutated p53 Ab-3 (OP 29-1) (103, 106, 107). Before performing the APAAP (105), slides with frozen sections were fixed in methanol and acetone and pretreated in a steamer (95 to 99°C). This was non-essential for p53 and Ki-67 but for hTERT and retinoic acid receptors nuclear staining in frozen sections essential (106, 107, 162). We determined p53 scores as described in 2.2. In quantitative presentation of antigen expression (p53, Ki-67, hTERT and retinoid receptors) by means of an immunoreactive score (IRS) we refer exclusively to the nuclear and / or nucleolar staining. We evaluated staining intensity (SI) and number of positive stained cells (PP) in the BCCs and in squamous cell epithelia of the tumor margin. The IRS was calculated by multiplication of SI and PP. In our immunohistochemical investigations the difference between IRS of p53 in tumor center (mean score value 7.9±3.4) was not significantly higher than in tumor margin (mean score value 5.8±4.2), $p=0.095$: Figure 5 and illustrated in Figure 6a (tumor center) and Figure 6c (tumor margin), cf. 2.3.2. p53 scores in T2-BCCs (8 primary tumors ≥2cm) were not higher than in T1-BCCs (17 primary tumors <2cm): mean score value 6.3±4.3 (T2) vs. 7.9±3.3 (T1), $p=0.328$. We tested the role of p53 scores investigated for prognosis in Kaplan-Meier curves (cf. 2.3.2). We divided all p53 scores (also Ki-67 scores and hTERT scores) into two groups (group 1: scores < mean value, group 2: scores ≥ mean value) and used the patients' up-to-date outcome as documented in our hospital. With all due reservation due to the many censored cases, we ascertain that BCCs of patients with higher p53 scores in tumor center tissues recurred later, almost significantly later, than BCCs of patients with lower scores in tumor center tissues (65±16 months vs. 23±6 months): Log-rank p=0.059, Figure 7a. However, patients with higher p53 scores in BCC tumor margin tissues did not relapse significantly but nevertheless earlier than patients with lower p53 scores in tumor margin tissues (36±6 months vs. 40±11 months): Log-rank p=0.622, Figure 7c.

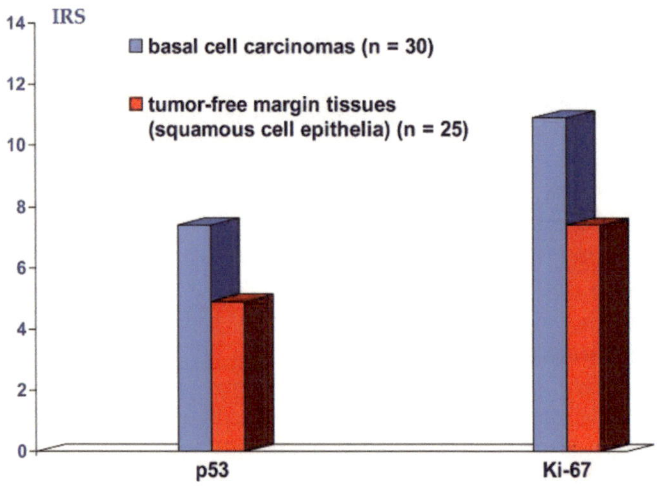

Fig. 5. IRS (immunoreactive scores, cf. 144, 145) mean values of expression of mutated p53 and of Ki-67 in basal cell carcinomas.

2.3.2 Marker Ki-67 in BCCs and BCC-free tumor margin tissues in comparison with p53

Some authors compared proof of p53 with expression of the proliferation marker Ki-67. Healy et al. (163) proved 71 BCC tissues immunohistochemically with p53 and Ki-67, 17 BCCs group 1 (patients without recurrence), 17 BCCs group 2-0 (patients who relapsed some time later) and 17 BCC relapses (group 2-R). p53 was demonstrated in 95% of each group. However, the authors (163) revealed significantly lower values of Ki-67 expression in BCCs in group 1 (mean value 12%) than in group 2-0 (mean value 25%) or group 2-R (mean value 22.5%): p=0.009. Barrett et al. (158) examined expression of p53, Ki-67 and PCNA in 27 basal cell carcinomas and compared them to histopathological BCC types. Expression of p53 and PCNA was higher in aggressive BCCs than in nonaggressive BCCs, and PCNA was higher than Ki-67. Chang et al. (100) tested 10 BCCs and detected both p53 and Ki-67 in all of them. The labeling index with Ki-67 was significantly lower than with p53: 12±7 vs. 50±17 (p <0.05). By contrast, in 20 BCCs Abdelsayed et al. (164) demonstrated higher marking with Ki-67 (mean value 51.25±6.06) and PCNA (mean value 52.25±7.57) than with p53 (mean value 31.75±9.02). Koseoglu et al. (161) also investigated the p53 level of 50 BCCs immunohistochemically in comparison with Ki-67 expression (anti-Ki-67 antibody clone Ki-88). They found significantly higher Ki-67 expression in p53 positive tissues (Ki-67 mean value 14.66) than in p53 negative tissues (Ki-67 mean value 8.37): p=0.019.

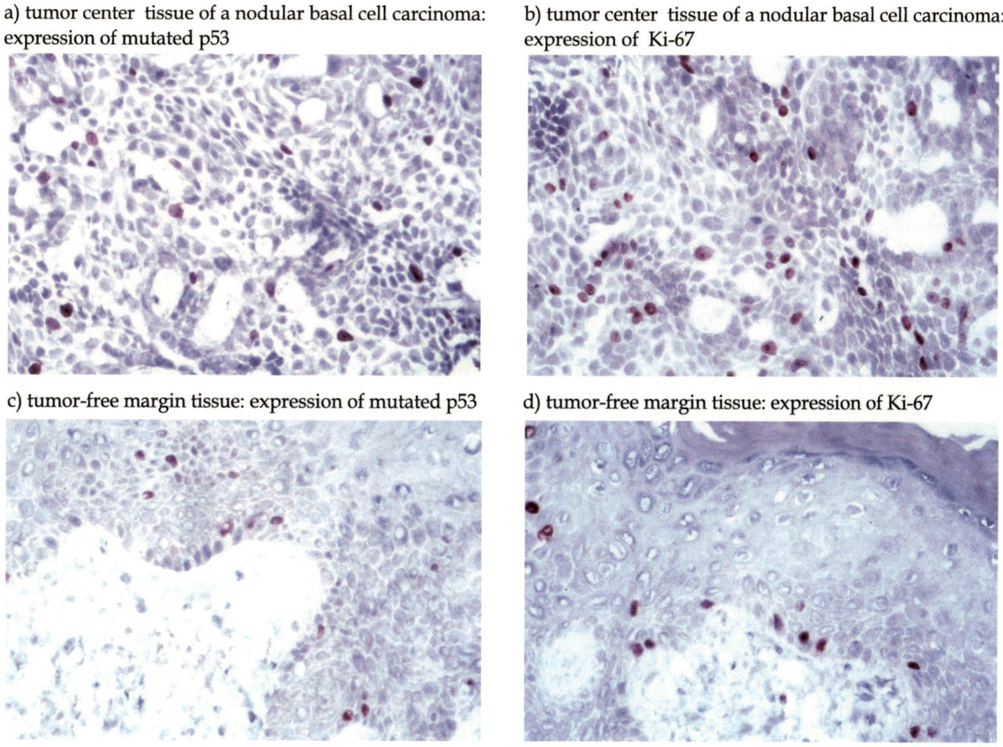

Fig. 6. Comparison of expression of p53 (a, c) and Ki-67 (b, d) in small frozen sections of BCCs (a, b) and in tumor margin tissues (c, d), magnification 400x.

We also compared Ki-67 scores with p53 scores in tumor center tissues and tumor-free margin tissues. To prove Ki-67 in small frozen sections we used a monoclonal mouse anti-human Ki-67 antibody (clone MIB-1) from DAKO (Denmark) (106, 107). As described under 2.2 and 2.3.1, nuclear staining scores were achieved with immunohistochemical APAAP (105). The Ki-67 mean score value in tumor center (10.9±2.5) was significantly higher than that in tumor margin (7.4±1.8), $p<0.05$: Figure 5, cf. 2.3.1. Our results with p53 and Ki-67 expression of tumor center and tumor margin tissues are displayed in Figure 6.

We tested the prognostic prediction of Ki-67 status (107) detected in our patients' tissues with BCCs in Kaplan-Meier curves. With all due reservation in view of the number of censored cases, patients with higher Ki-67 scores in tumor center tissues suffered BCC recurrence (not significantly) later (Log-rank $p=0.560$) than patients with lower Ki-67 scores (56±16 months, higher scores, vs. 27±7 months, lower scores): Figure 7b. In contrast, patients with higher Ki-67-scores in tumor margin tissues did not relapse significantly earlier (Log-rank $p=0.321$) than patients with lower Ki-67-scores (35±5 months, higher scores, vs. 48±13 months, lower scores): Figure 7d.

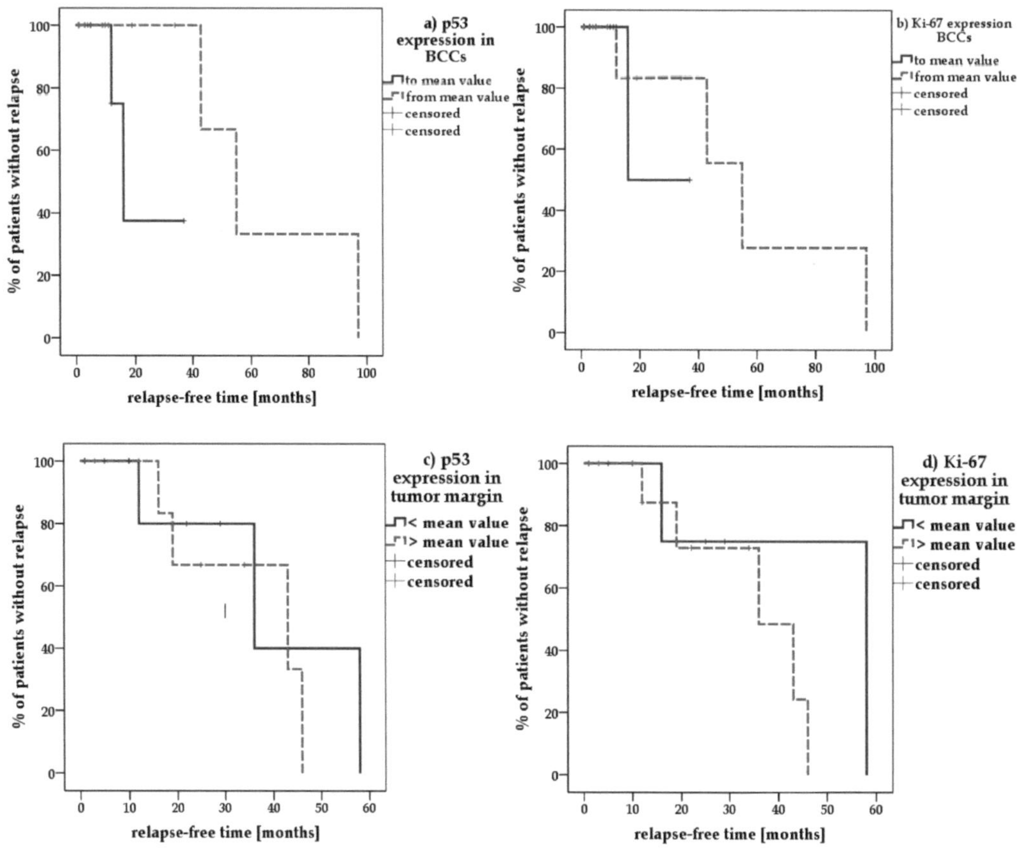

Fig. 7. Kaplan-Meier curves for p53 expression (a, c) and Ki-67 expression (b, d) in BCC tumor center tissues (a, b) and in tumor margin tissues (c, d).

2.4 The biology of telomerase

In 1984 Blackburn and Greider discovered telomerase in a single-celled ciliate *Tetrahymena* (165, 166), a ribonucleoprotein enzyme. The enzyme is of universal importance for cell proliferation. Telomerase replaces the mitotic loss of telomeres at chromosome ends with telomeric substitutes. This abrogates the limited cell division potential (the Hayflick limit). Hayflick and Moorhead (167) observed limited cell division in fibroblast cultures. Activation of telomerase occurs during embryogenesis (168, 169). In normal somatic tissues with a limited replicative potential telomerase activity can be demonstrated only in traces or not at all (170 to 172). Activation of telomerase can be found inside cells with proliferative potential such as stem cells, in strongly regenerative cells, and in dermal cells of hair follicles (169, 171 to 175). Telomerase can be activated by UVB in seriously sun-exposed skin (10, 64). It may also be detected in benign proliferative lesions (174) or after activation in cells of inflammatory reactions (170, 172, 174, 176 to 178). Reactivation of telomerase also occurs in carcinogenesis (179, 180), as was illustrated by Ueda et al. (64) (Figure 1, 1.1). It is an essential step for cancer immortalization and cancer progression (172, 180).

However not until Kim et al. (168) developed the polymerase chain reaction based telomeric repeat amplification protocol in 1994 (TRAP assay) was it possible to detect telomerase in greater numbers in unfixed tissues. Since then, a great number of tissues, particularly from cancer, have been investigated for telomerase activity as the reviews by Shay and Bacchetti (181) and Dhaene et al. (182) demonstrate.

2.4.1 Activation of telomerase in tumor center and tumor margin tissues of BCCs

The results of telomerase activity in BCCs and tumor-free adjacent tissues have been summarized. The portion of 203 specimens with evidence of telomerase detected with the TRAP assay (168) amounted to an average of 87%, varying between 20 and 100% (64, 103, 104, 183 to 189). Table 1 sums up telomerase activity of BCCs and tumor-free adjacent tissues. To discriminate between BCC center tissue and tumor-free margin tissue Taylor et al. (183) and Ueda et al. (64) introduced proof of telomerase activity. They found clearly less telomerase activity in tumor margin tissue than in the tumor center: BCC margin tissues with 67% and 39% vs. 95% and 85% of BCC center tissues.

References	**telomerase positive in tumor center tissues**	**telomerase positive in tumor margin tissues**
Taylor et al., 1996 (183)	73/77 (95%)	38/57 (67%)
Ueda et al., 1997 (64)	11/13 (85%)	11/28 (39%)
Parris et al., 1999 (184)	10/13 (77%)	
Wu et al., 1999 (185)	10/11 (91%)	
Kim et al., 2000 (186)	1/ 5 (20%)	
Chen et al., 2001 (187)	22/22 (100%)	
Boldrini et al., 2003 (188)	15/20 (75%)	
Fabricius et al.,2003 (103) and 2006 (104)	26/30 (87%)	9/25 (36%)
Saleh et al., 2007 (189)	9/12 (75%)	
altogether	**177/203 (87%)**	**58/110 (53%)**

The extinction values of the PCR-ELISA were negative at 0-150 mOD, 1+ = 150-450 mOD, 2+ = 450-750 mOD 3+, = 750-1050 mOD and 4+ above1050 mOD (102, 103).

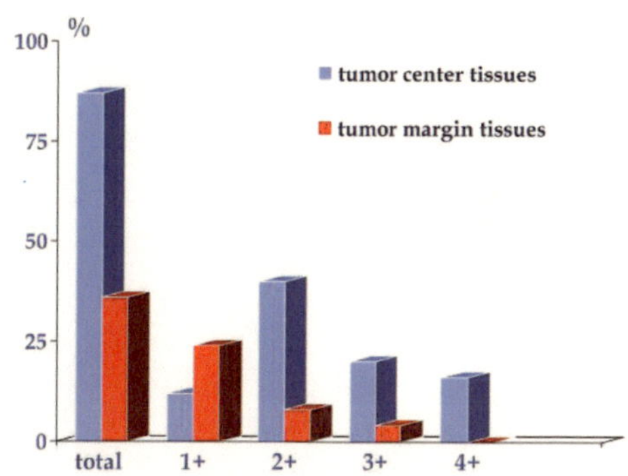

Fig. 8. Telomerase activity in BCCs and in tumor-free margin tissues (103, 104)

Table 1. The frequency of telomerase activity (detected with the TRAP assay) in basal cell carcinomas and their tumor-free margin tissues.

Like Taylor et al. (183) and Ueda et al. (64), we found significantly higher telomerase activity in 26/30 (87%) of BCC tumor center tissues (mean value 661±388 mOD) than in 9/25 (36%) histopathologically tumor-free tumor margin tissues (mean value 187±233 mOD) (103, 104). As we proved telomerase activity semiquantitatively with a PCR-ELISA (Telo TAGGG Telomerase PCR and PCR-ELISA plus, Roche Diagnostics, Germany) we were able to be somewhat more precise: the mean value of telomerase activation in BCC tumor tissues was significantly higher than in tumor margin tissues: $p<0.001$. In contrast, telomerase activation in T2 tumors (mean value 564±225 mOD) did not differ significantly from telomerase activation in T1 tumors (mean value 709±446 mOD): p=0.783. In Figure 8, our study on telomerase activation in tumor center and tumor margin has been compiled according to extinction values.

We tested whether the telomerase examined in BCCs or tumor margin tissues has prognostic relevance (103, 104). We divided all measured values of telomerase (PCR-ELISA) and divided the patients into two groups, group 1: < mean value and group 2: ≥ mean value, and used the patients' up-to-date outcome as documented in our hospital. In Kaplan-Meier curves of tumors and tumor margin tissues, patients with higher telomerase activity suffered recurrence earlier than patients with lower telomerase activity but not significantly: tumor center: 36±9 vs. 97±0 months (Log-rank: p=0.100), tumor margin: 19±1 vs. 42±6 months (Log-rank: p=0.141): Figure 9.

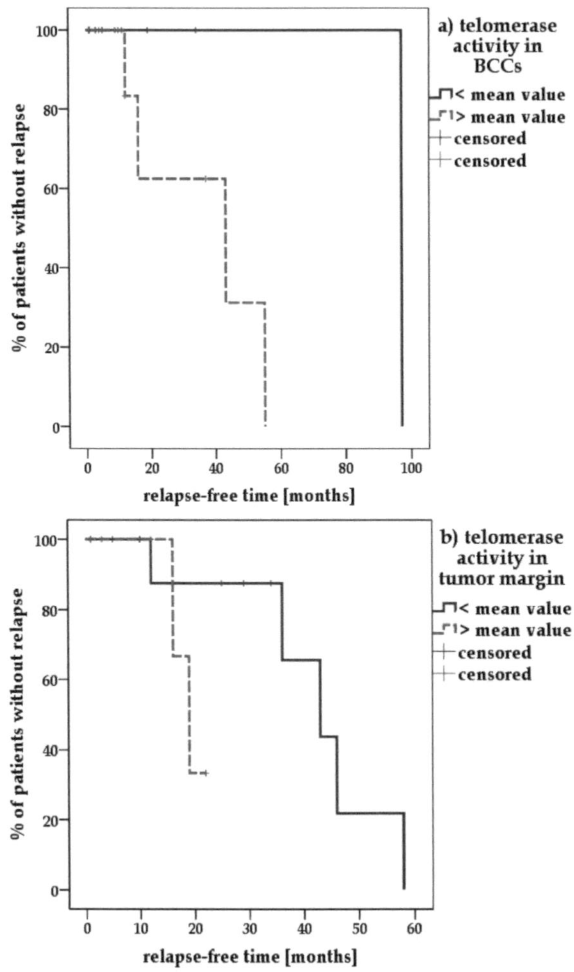

Fig. 9. Comparison of Kaplan-Meier curve for telomerase activity in BCCs (a) and tumor-free margin tissues (b).

Detection of telomerase activity in unfixed BCC tissues and tumor margin tissues can corroborate, with due reservation in view of the censored cases, histopathological and clinical assessment of risk of recurrence.

2.4.2 Expression of hTERT in tumor center and tumor margin tissues of BCCs

hTERT (human telomerase reverse transcriptase) is a catalytic subunit and a component of telomerase (171, 190, 191). Proof of hTERT protein can be carried out both in unfixed and in fixed tissue and facilitates the localization of telomerase activity. The detectable evidence of the hTERT protein or hTERT mRNA might, however, not always mirror detectable telomerase activity (171).

Saleh et al. (189) used proof of hTERT to differentiate between BCCs of differing size and histopathological type. They determined hTERT in all of 12 BCCs, with no significant difference between mRNA hTERT by RTq-PCR in BCCs of different size: mean value BCCs <9 mm 0.458 vs. mean value BCCs ≥9 mm 0.478. In tumor-free margin tissues of larger BCCs the authors (189) found a somewhat lower, non-significant expression of hTERT mRNA (BCC <9 mm mean value 0.160, BCC ≥9 mm 0.119). hTERT expression of superficial BCCs (n=5), however, was significantly lower ($p<0.05$) than that of nodular BCCs (n=7): tumor center mean value 0.305 vs. 0.525 and tumor-free margin 0.094 vs. 0.172. With senior patients (≥65 years of age, n=6) Saleh et al. (189) succeeded in determining non-significant hTERT expression in tumors and tumor-free margin tissues that was lower than that in younger patients (<65 years of age, n=6): tumor center mean value 0.343 vs. 0.593 and tumor margin 0.104 vs. 0.175. Proof of hTERT was also established by Hu et al. (192) and Park et al. (98) for evaluating BCCs. Hu et al. (192) examined 62 fresh skin tissues in RT-PCR. They compared hTERT with TPI (another protein component of telomerase) and with hTR, an RNA component of telomerase (171). Part of their study (192) was the investigation of 4 BCCs, all of which expressed hTERT, TPI and 3 / 4 hTR. Park et al. (98) demonstrated hTERT 2+ to 3+ in 8 / 10 BCCs in paraffin sections with anti-hTERT antibody from Calbiochem (USA, Ab-2). Ogoshi et al. (193) used in situ hybridization to prove hTERT and confirmed its occurrence in 93% (14/15) of BCCs.

Attia et al. (194) introduced the anti-hTERT antibody code NCL-hTERT (clone 44F12, Novocastra, UK) for evidence of immunohistochemical hTERT in normal tissues such as in photo-exposed skin. The authors succeeded in proving hTERT (1+ to 3+) in 80% of the epidermis of photo-aged subjects. hTERT was expressed in normal skin in the basal layer and in some supra-basal layers, as well as in hair follicles (cf. telomerase activity in hair follicles: 173 to 175).

In our study with small frozen sections we used eleven anti-hTERT antibodies to detect and localize hTERT expression in 25 BCC tumor tissues and 25 tumor margin tissues (107). Previously we had employed the same antibodies to examine squamous cell carcinomas and SCC tumor margin tissues (106). Before performing APAAP (105), slides were fixed in methanol and acetone and pretreated in a steamer (95 to 99°C). As described in detail in our first study (106), this pretreatment was essential for hTERT nuclear staining in frozen sections. The most prominent immunohistochemical effects were achieved with anti-hTERT antibody code NCL-hTERT (clone 44F12, Novocastra, UK), which was also used by Attia et al. (194) for hTERT detection in sun exposed skin. This antibody was classified later in the paper by Wu et al. (195) as an antibody against nucleolin. We expanded our investigation and incorporated an anti-nucleolin antibody to clarify this issue (106, 107). On the basis of our peptide absorption studies (106) and in agreement with many authors we think that this antibody clone 44F12 Novocastra identifies hTERT. We compared the results of BCCs (107) with antibody Calbiochem, USA, code 582005 and others, and determined the hTERT scores as described in 2.2 and 2.3.1. In the quantitative presentation of antigen expression we refer exclusively to the nuclear and / or nucleolar staining. We evaluated staining intensity (SI) and the number of positive stained cells (PP) in the BCCs and in squamous cell epithelia of the tumor margin. The IRS was calculated by multiplication of SI and PP (144, 145).

Our immunohistochemical proof of hTERT is predominantly localized in tumor and in squamous cell epithelia of BCCs and BCC tumor-free margin tissues. hTERT scores with a polyclonal antibody (Calbiochem/USA, code 582005, Ab 1) and with a monoclonal antibody (Novocastra/UK, code NCL-hTERT, clone 44F12, Ab 2) are significantly lower in the tumor margin (mean score values Ab 1 5.4±3.3 and Ab 2 7.0±2.9) than in tumor center (mean score values Ab 1 9.4±4.9 and Ab 2 9.0±3.9): $p=0.002$ and $p=0.011$ (107). In Figures 10 and 11, hTERT expression is demonstrated with two antibodies. Proof of hTERT expression now and then differs from telomerase activity.

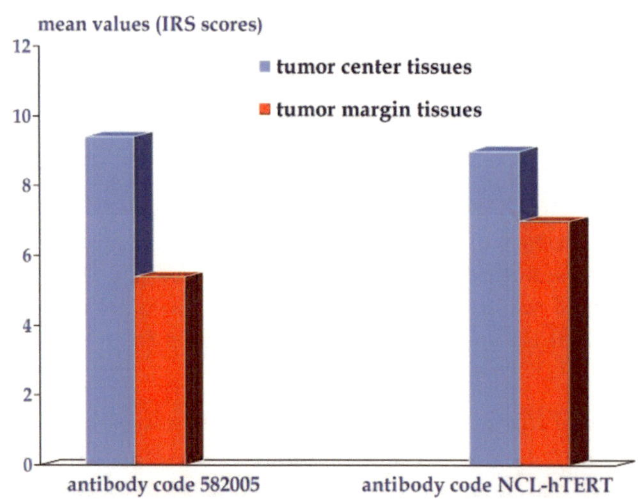

Fig. 10. Mean values of immunoreactive score (cf. 144, 145) with two anti-hTERT antibodies (Calbiochem/USA and Novocastra/UK).

a) tumor center tissue of a nodular basal cell carcinoma (telomerase activity 3+), Ab 1

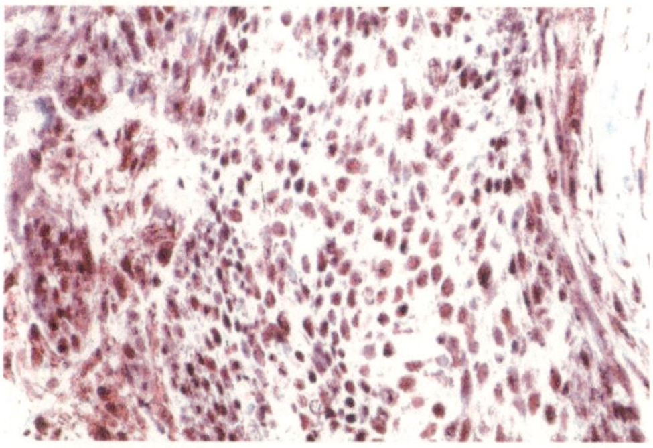

b) tumor center tissue of a nodular basal cell carcinoma (telomerase activity 3+), Ab 2

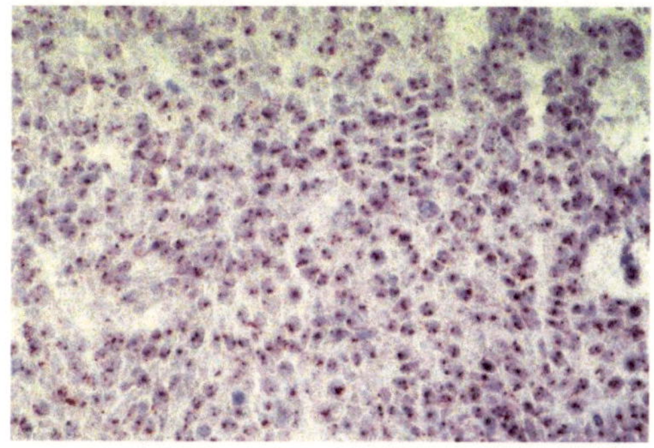

c) tumor center tissue of a mixed nodular-sclerodermiform BCC (telomerase activity 1+), Ab 1

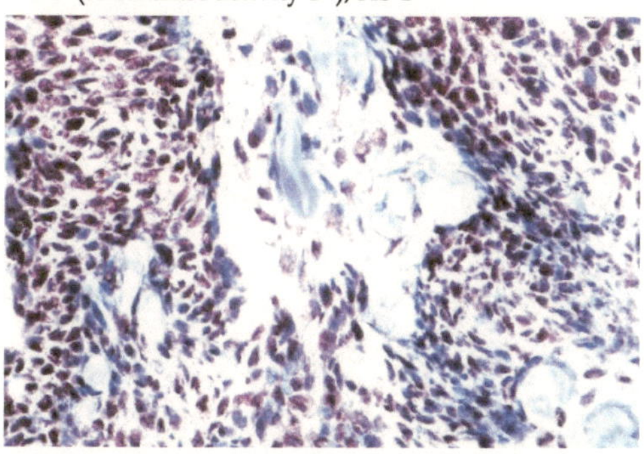

d) tumor center tissue of a mixed nodular-sclerodermiform BCC (telomerase activity 1+), Ab 2

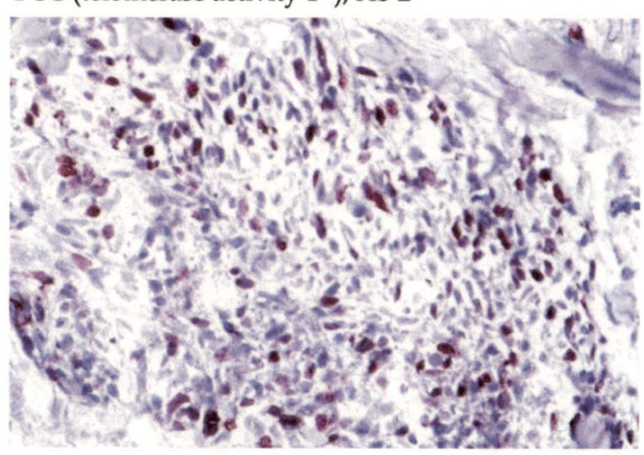

e) tumor margin tissue of a nodular BCC (telomerase activity 1+), Ab 1

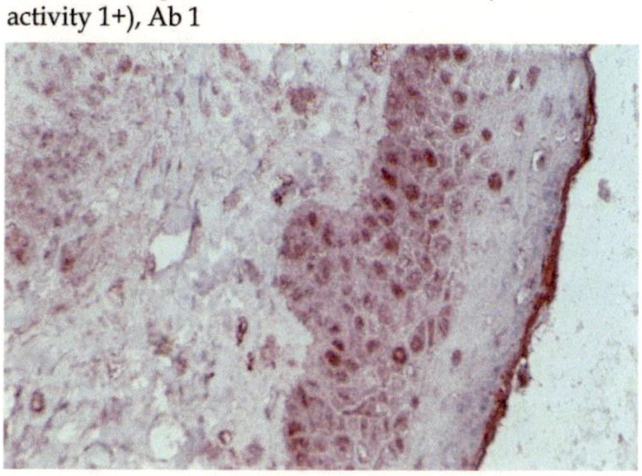

f) tumor margin tissue of a nodular BCC (telomerase activity 1+), Ab 2

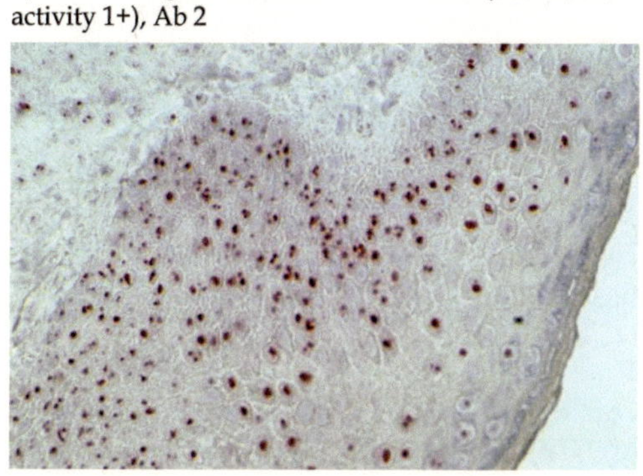

Fig. 11. Comparison of hTERT expression with two anti-hTERT antibodies: polyclonal antibody code 582005, Ab 1 (a, c and e) and monoclonal antibody code NCL-hTERT, clone 44F12, Ab 2 (b, d and f), magnification 400x.

Kaplan-Meier curves indicate that proof of hTERT does not reveal the further course of the disease. We divided all hTERT scores into two groups (group 1: < mean value, group 2: ≥ mean value) and related them with the patients' up-to-date outcome as documented in our hospital. With the caveat that there were many censored cases, it can be said that patients with higher hTERT scores in tumor center tissues relapsed earlier than patients with lower hTERT scores in tumor center tissues: antibody code 582005 (Ab 1): 43±8 months vs. 70±31 months, Log-rank p=0.539, Figure 12a; antibody code NCL-hTERT (Ab 2): 42±9 months vs.

77±25 months, Log-rank p=0.387, Figure 12b. However, patients with higher hTERT scores in BCC tumor-free margin tissues did not relapse earlier than those with lower hTERT scores in tumor-free margin tissues: antibody code 582005 (Ab 1): 43±9 months vs. 30±9 months, Log-rank p=0.230, Figure 12c; antibody code NCL-hTERT (Ab 2): 39±5 months vs. 32±5 months, Log-rank p=0.686, Figure 12d.

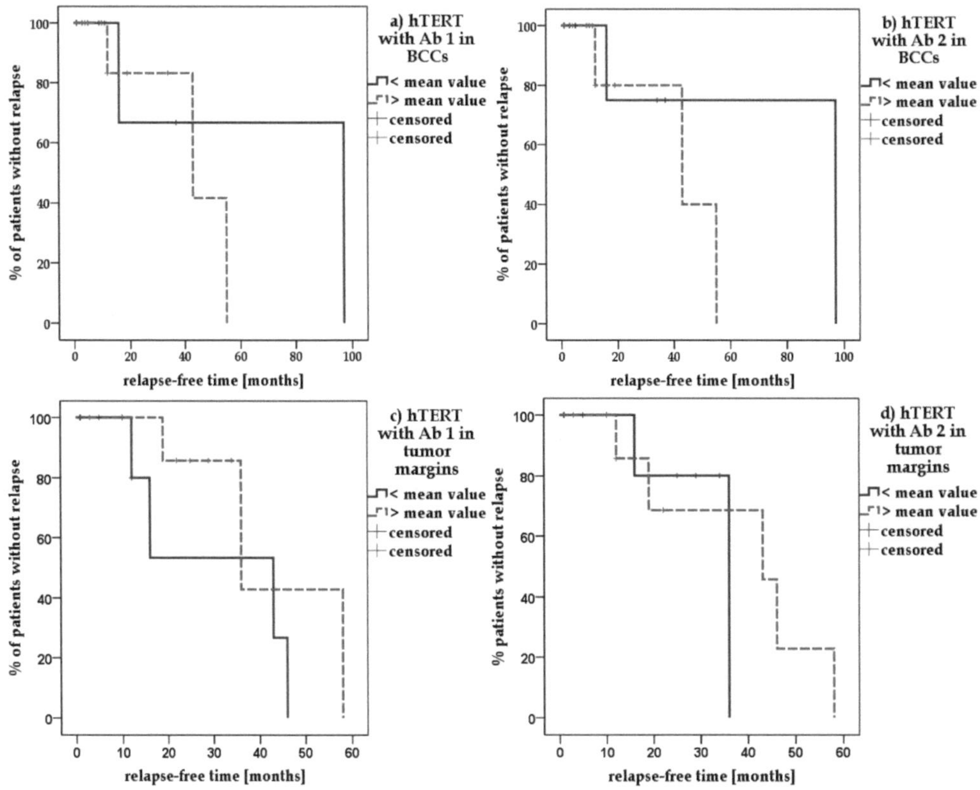

Fig. 12. Kaplan-Meier curves of hTERT expression in BCCs (a and b) and tumor-free margin tissues (c and d): Ab 1 = polyclonal antibody code 582005, Ab 2 = monoclonal antibody code NCL-hTERT.

Our hTERT results in tissues from patients with basal cell carcinoma (107) verify the value of hTERT in localizing the cells in which telomerase is activated (2.4.1). Although we identified differences between eleven antibodies (106, 107), we succeeded in detecting hTERT expression primarily in tumor cells and in squamous epithelia cells (Figure 11) after pretreatment of frozen sections in the steamer. We applied the same unfixed tissues for proof of telomerase activity and for hTERT expression. As McKenzie et al. (171) had already discovered, our detection of hTERT might not always mirror detectable telomerase activity (Figure 11, a to f). Kyo et al. (196) arrived at the same conclusion that hTERT did not always correlate with telomerase activity of the various cell types.

Given our previous observations, we decided to evaluate only nuclear or nucleolar expression of hTERT although some antibodies also displayed cytoplasmic staining (106, 107). It must be mentioned, however, that investigations of gynaecologic carcinomatous tissues by Kyo et al. (196) established proof of both hTERT and high levels of telomerase after the isolation of cytoplasms, so further evaluation for immunohistochemical proof of hTERT is warranted. Taken together, both telomerase and hTERT may be useful as biomarkers in predicting chemotherapeutic effects (197).

3. Biomarkers for chemoprevention of basal cell carcinomas

Given frequent BCC recurrence and field cancerization in tumor-free margin tissues, several studies were launched to investigate the efficacy of chemoprevention in patients with a basal cell carcinoma. The best and primary prevention of basal cell carcinomas is reduction of the most important risk factor, exposure to strong sunlight from childhood (11, 12, 15, 18, 21, 23, 39, 52, 198). The use of agents that inhibit the noxious influence of UV light (199) could therefore be the most effective preventive method. In addition, there have been many studies applying retinoids (topical and oral / systemic) to suppress the emergence of basal cell carcinomas (200 to 207) and thus influence field cancerization of skin and tumor surroundings (59 to 63) to prevent new tumors and / or tumor recurrences. For immunosuppressed patients, chemoprevention is particularly important (63, 198, 208 to 210). After chemoprevention proved to be unsuccessful in most studies, receptor-selective retinoids such as tazarotene were tried out (211 to 218). Tazarotene is selective for retinoic acid receptors RARβ and RARγ. Thus Bianchi et al. (217) successfully applied tazarotene-gel preoperatively for small superficial and nodular BCCs. This was not successful on keratotic BCCs with high p53 expression, and they were operated afterwards. Crucial for effective retinoic acid chemoprevention and / or therapy is the expression of RAR- and RXR-receptors (218, 219), as was demonstrated by So et al. (220). So et al. consider tazarotene to be the most appropriate agent to date for chemoprevention of BCCs.

In addition to synthesis of suitable agents it is essential to search for suitable biomarkers to improve prevention (19), and markers such as p53, Ki-67 or telomerase (2.3 and 2.4) merit consideration along with other genetic markers. Intermediate markers are needed in particular for chemoprevention trials (204). To determine a preliminary endpoint, genetic, cellular, biochemical and immunological surrogate biomarkers - surrogate endpoint markers (SEBs) - are being used and validated so that BCC chemoprevention can be evaluated before a recurrence becomes evident (204, 221 to 225). Orlandi et al. (225) employed the markers Ki-67, p53, apoptosis-index, RARα, RARβ and RARγ before and after tazarotene therapy of 30 BCCs. Expression of Ki-67 was significantly reduced after therapy compared with controls (11% vs. 29%, $p<0.001$). Expression of p53 was unchanged after therapy. In comparison with controls, however, evidence of apoptotic cells was significantly higher after therapy (4.5% vs. 1%, $p<0.001$). While expression of RARα and RARγ was not changed through therapy, expression of receptor RARβ was distinctly higher. In our model investigations with cell cultures of oral squamous cell carcinomas, telomerase proved to be a suitable biomarker before and after retinoid therapy (162). Verification with BCCs is yet to follow.

Examination of RAR receptors (retinoic acid receptors) and RXR receptors (retinoid X receptors) on BCCs might indicate why most studies do not show any differences between therapy and placebo groups. Using immunohistochemical methods, Kamradt and Reichrath (226) investigated expression of RAR receptors in frozen sections of 15 basal cell carcinomas: RARα was most evident (3 +), RARγ a little weaker (2 +) and RARβ scanty (0 to 1 +). This corroborates studies by Hartmann et al. (227). In comparison with SCCs of the skin, the authors determined RAR receptors of 28 BCCs by RTq-PCR. Measured values of this study were also lowest for RARβ-mRNA (7.91 x 10^{-5}) and distinctly higher for RARα (1.97 x 10^{-3}) and RARγ (1.25 x 10^{-2}).

Approximately comparable with regard to tumor-free margin tissues are immunohistochemical investigations by Reichrath et al. (228) on normal skin RAR- and RXR receptors of 12 male volunteers. Expression of RARα was most distinctly detectable, among other things, in epidermal keratinocytes (5 +) and in hair follicle keratinocytes (5 +). Expression of RARγ was distinct in epidermal keratinocytes (2 +) and in hair follicles (3 +), but expression of RARβ was found in traces only (0 to 1 +). All three RXR receptors RXRα, RXRβ and RXRγ were distinctly expressed (2 +, mostly 3 +) in both of these cell types.

We therefore tested as well for expression of RAR and RXR receptors in small frozen sections of BCCs with immunohistochemical APAAP (105). After fixing pretreatment in a steamer, which was essential in our study for clear and strong nuclear receptor detection in frozen sections (162, cf. 106, 107), we applied antibodies from Santa Cruz / USA (anti-RARα, code sc-551; anti-RXRβ1, code sc-556 and anti-RXRγ, code sc-555), from Abcam / USA (anti-RARβ, code ab15515) and from Abnova / USA (anti-RXRα, code H00006256 M01). Other antibodies were less suitable for our frozen sections. In our study the anti-RARγ antibody was inappropriate (162). Evaluation succeeded with immunoreactive scores (IRS) as described with p53, Ki-67 and hTERT (2.3.1, 2.3.2 and 2.4.2). For control we investigated tissues with comparable localization from BCC-free patients. Figure 13 summarizes mean score values for

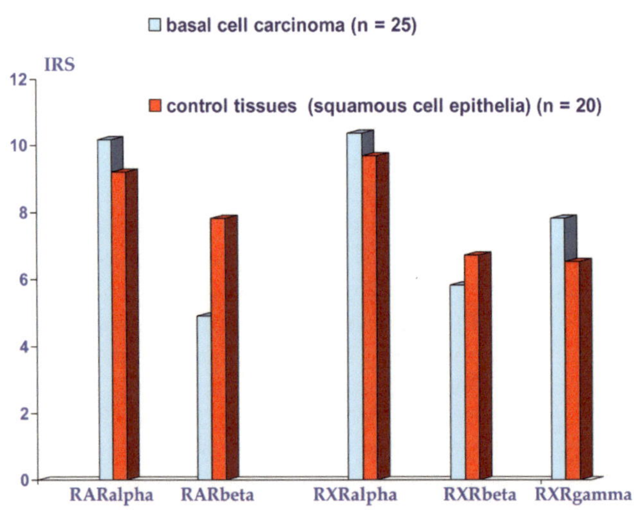

Fig. 13. Immunoreactive scores (IRS, cf. 144, 145) of expression for RAR and RXR receptors in small frozen sections of BCCs and control tissues (mean values).

expression of RAR and RXR receptors. In agreement with Kamradt and Reichrath (226) and with Hartmann (227) we were able to detect all receptors tested in BCCs in similar levels as in control tissues. RARβ expression in BCCs had the lowest value (mean score value 4.92±1.81), followed by RXRβ (mean score value 5.83±1.76), RXRγ (mean score value 7.83±2.36), RARα (mean score value 10.17±2.02) and RXRα (mean score value 10.38±2.14). Expression of RARβ was almost significantly lower in BCCs than in control tissues (p=0.056). The expression of the remaining receptors in BCCs and control tissues did not differ statistically: p=0.586 (RARα), p=0.862 (RXRα), p=0.863 (RXRβ) and p= 0.871 (RXRγ).

Our results suggest that the increase of RARβ in the context of a chemoprevention might give us valuable information as a surrogate end point biomarker for the success of therapy in chemoprevention, as was previously demonstrated by Orlandi et al. (225). Figures 14a to 14e illustrate expression patterns of receptors in small frozen sections of basal cell carcinomas.

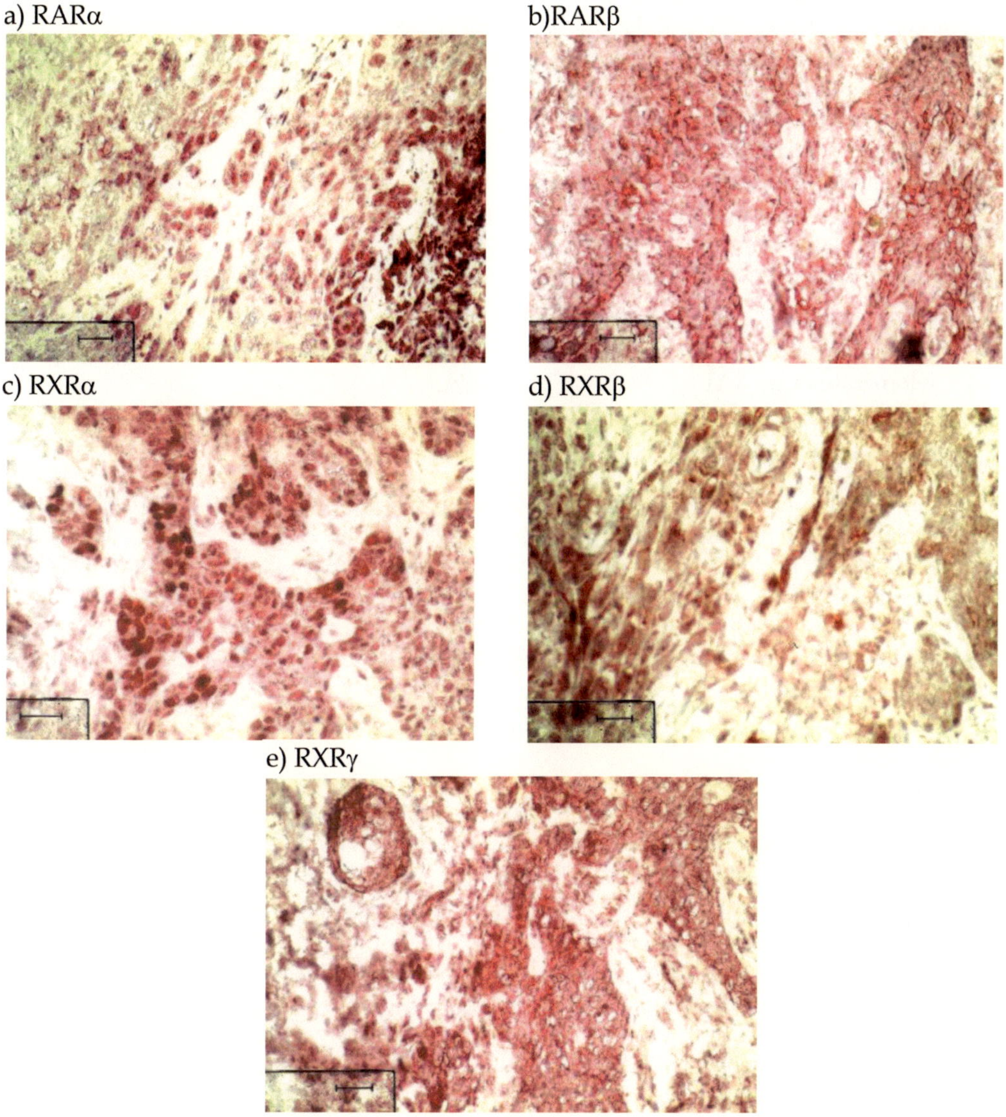

Fig. 14. Expression of retinoic acid receptors (RAR) and retinoid X receptors (RXR) of a nodular BCC (frozen sections); bars 20 μm.

4. Conclusion

Immunohistochemical application of Ber-Ep4 (85 to 88) is particularly appropriate for histopathological differentiation between SCCs of the skin and basal cell carcinomas. When examined with immunohistochemical methods, adhesion molecules CD44v6 and U36 (CD44v6-chimera) give clear evidence for spreading of BCCs (Figure 4) and for the absence of tumor in tumor margins (91 to 96, 134 to 138, cf. 131 to 133). Radionuclide-labeled antibodies developed against oral squamous cell carcinomas (146 to 156, 229, 230) might also be applied in the diagnosis and therapy of patients with BCC.

It is important for prognostic purposes to make a clear distinction between smaller T1-BCCs and larger T2-BCCs (cf. 2. and Figure 2). Clinical classification into aggressive and less aggressive BCCs confirmed by histopathology can be supported, among other things, by markers p53 (101, 103, 121 to 124, 157 to 161), bcl-2 (81, 100, 122), Ki-67 (100, 106, 107, 158, 161) and by the apoptotic index (124). The markers Ki-67 and p53 can impart supplementary information and are important for histopathological diagnosis with regard to making a clinical judgement of the consequences of "tumor-free margin". Representation of telomerase activity in unfixed tumor margin tissues (64, 103, 104, 183), and not so much immunohistochemical proof of hTERT, (98, 107, 189, 192) can contribute to a better diagnostic assessment of tumor-free margins and may indicate early recurrence.

The high proportion of BCC recurrences is a challenge to develop better selective agents for chemoprevention and to support them with appropriate biomarkers such as Ki-67, apoptotic index, telomerase or by RARβ (199, 214, 225, cf. 162).

5. Acknowledgements

We are indebted to Prof. Swen O. Warnaar, CENTOCOR B.V. (Leiden/The Netherlands) for the generous gift of the MoAb U36 and MoAb E48 used in our studies. At our hospital Charité we thank Prof. Gustav-Paul Wildner for the histopathological evaluation of the small frozen sections and Mrs. Catherine Aubel for language help and editing. We thank Mrs. Ute Kruse-Boitschenko for her technical aid in the laboratory and Mr. Franz Hafner for the photo scanning. Our study was supported by grants from the Berlin Sparkasse Foundation for Medicine.

6. References

[1] Krüger, K.; Blume-Peytavi, U. & Orfanos, C.E. (1999). Basal cell carcinoma possibly originates from the outer root sheath and/or the bulge region of the vellus hair follicle. *Arch Dermatol Res* 291: 253-259

[2] Lacour, J. (2002). Carcinogenesis of basal cell carcinomas: genetics and molecular mechanisms. *Br J Dermatol* 146: 17-19

[3] Tilli, C.M.; Van Steensel, M.A.; Krekels, G.A.; Neumann, H.A. & Ramaekers, F.C. (2005). Molecular aetiology and pathogenesis of basal cell carcinoma. *Br J Dermatol* 152: 1108-1124

[4] Crowson, A.N. (2006). Basal cell carcinoma: biology, morphology and clinical implications. *Mod Pathol* 19: S127-S147

[5] Donovan, J. (2009). Review of the hair follicle origin hypothesis for basal cell carcinoma. *Dermatol Surg* 35: 1311-1323

[6] Harris, P.J.; Takebe, N. & Ivy, S.P. (2010). Molecular conversations and the development of the hair follicle and basal cell carcinoma. *Cancer Prev Res (Phila)* 3: 1217-1221
[7] Zackheim, H.S. (1964). Comparative cutaneous carcinogenesis in the rat. Differential response to the application of anthramine, methylcholanthrene, and dimethylbenzanthracene. *Oncology* 17: 236-246
[8] Bajdik, C.; Gallagher, R.; Astrakianakis, G.; Hill, G.; Fincham, S. & McLean, D. (1996). Non-solar ultraviolet radiation and the risk of basal and squamous cell skin cancer. *Br J Cancer* 73: 1612-1614
[9] Nishigori, C. (2000). UV-induced DNA damage in carcinogenesis and its repair. J Dermatol Sci 23: S41-S44
[10] Ueda, M. (2000). Telomerase in cutaneous carcinogenesis. *J Dermatol Sci* 23: S37-S40
[11] Armstrong, B. & Kricker, A. (2001). The epidemiology and UV induced skin cancer. *J Photochem Photobiol B* 63: 8-18
[12] Corona, R.; Dogliotti, E.; D'Errico, M.; Sera, F.; Iavarone, I.; Baliva, G.; Chinni, L.; Gobello, T.; Mazzanti, C.; Puddu, P. & Pasquini, P. (2001). Risk factors for basal cell carcinoma in a mediterranean population - role of recreational sun exposure early in life. *Arch Dermatol* 137: 1162-1168; comment 1239-1240
[13] Tran, H.; Chen, K. & Shumack, S. (2003). Epidemiology and aetiology of basal cell carcinoma. *Br J Dermatol* 149: 50-52
[14] Ramos, J.; Villa, J.; Ruiz, A.; Armstrong, R. & Matta, J. (2004). UV dose determines key characteristics of nonmelanoma skin cancer. *Cancer Epidemiol Biomarkers Prev* 13: 2006-2011
[15] Boukamp, P. (2005). [UV-induced skin cancer: similarities—variations.] Durch UV-Strahlung induzierte Hauttumore: Gemeinsamkeiten - Unterschiede. *J Dtsch Dermatol Ges* 3: 493-503
[16] Boukamp, P. (2005). Non-melanoma skin cancer: what drives tumor development and progression? *Carcinogenesis* 26: 1657-1667
[17] Nindl, I.; Gottschling, M. & Stockfleth, E. (2007). Human papillomaviruses and non-melanoma skin cancer: basic virology and clinical manifestations. *Dis Markers* 23: 247-259
[18] Rigel, D.S. (2008). Cutaneous ultraviolet exposure and its relationship to the development of skin cancer. *J Am Acad Dermatol* 58: S129-S132
[19] Greinert, R. (2009). Skin cancer: new markers for better prevention. *Pathobiology* 76: 64-81
[20] Kyrgidis, A.; Vahtsevanos, K.; Tzellos, T.G.; Xirou, P.; Kitikidou, K.; Antoniades, K.; Zouboulis, C.C. & Triaridis, S. (2010). New concepts for basal cell carcinoma. Demographic, clinical, histological risk factors, and biomarkers. A systematic review of evidence regarding risk for tumor development, susceptibility for second primary and recurrence. *J Surg Res* 159: 545-556
[21] Kütting, B. & Drexler, H. (2010). UV-induced skin cancer at workplace and evidence-based prevention. *Int Arch Occup Environ Health* 83: 843-854
[22] Patel, R.V.; Frankel, A. & Goldenberg, G. (2011). An update on nonmelanoma skin cancer. *J Clin Aesthet Dermatol* 4: 20-27
[23] Göppner, D. & Leverkus, M. (2011). Basal cell carcinoma: from the molecular understanding of the pathogenesis to targeted therapy of progressive disease. *J Skin Cancer,* Volume 2011, Article ID 650258, 8 pages

[24] Golitz, L.E.; Norris, D.A.; Luekens, C.A. Jr & Charles, D.M. (1980). Nevoid basal cell carcinoma syndrome. Multiple basal cell carcinomas of the palms after radiation therapy. *Arch Dermatol* 116: 1159-1163

[25] Howell, J.B. (1984). Nevoid basal cell carcinoma syndrome. Profile of genetic and environmental factors in oncogenesis. *J Am Acad Dermatol* 11: 98-104

[26] Gorlin, R.J. (1987). Nevoid basal-cell carcinoma syndrome. *Medicine (Baltimore)* 66 :98-113

[27] Miller, S.J. (1995). Etiology and pathogenesis of basal cell carcinoma. *Clin Dermatol* 13: 527-536

[28] Heagerty, A.; Smith, A.; English, J.; Lear, J.; Perkins, W.; Bowers, B.; Jones, P.; Gilford, J.; Alldersea, J.; Fryer, A. & Strange, R.C. (1996). Susceptibility to multiple cutaneous basal cell carcinomas: significant interactions between glutathione S-transferase GSTM1 genotypes, skin type and male gender. *Br J Cancer* 73: 44-48

[29] Lear, J.; Tan, B.; Smith, A.; Bowers, W.; Jones, P.; Heagerty, A.; Strange, R. & Fryer; A. (1997). Basal cell carcinoma. Risk factors for basal cell carcinoma in the UK: case-control study in 806 patients. *J R Soc Med* 90: 371-374

[30] Wallberg, P.; Kaaman, T. & Lindberg, M.(1998). Multiple basal cell carcinomas. A clinical evaluation of risk factors. *Acta Derm Venereol* 78: 127-129

[31] Fusenig, N. & Boukamp, P. (1998). Multiple stages and genetic alterations in immortalization, malignant transformation, and tumor progression of human skin keratinocytes. *Mol Carcinog* 23: 144-158

[32] Ramachandran, S.; Lear, J.T.; Ramsay, H.; Smith, A.G.; Bowers, B.; Hutchinson, P.E.; Jones, P.W.; Fryer, A.A. & Strange, R.C. (1999). Presentation with multiple cutaneous basal cell carcinomas: association of glutathione S-transferase and cytochrome P450 genotypes with clinical phenotype. *Cancer Epidemiol Biomarkers Prev* 8: 61-67

[33] Sarasin, A. (1999). The molecular pathways of ultraviolet-induced carcinogenesis. *Mutat Res* 428: 5-10

[34] Ramachandran, S.; Fryer, A.; Smith, A.; Lear, J.; Bowers, B.; Griffiths, C.; Jones, P. & Strange, R. (2000). Basal cell carcinoma. Tumor clustering is associated with incresed accrual in high risk subgroups. *Cancer* 89: 1012-1018

[35] Ramachandran, S.; Fryer, A.A.; Lovatt, T.; Lear, J.; Smith, A.G. & Strange, R.C. (2001). Susceptibility and modifier genes in cutaneous basal cell carcinomas and their associations with clinical phenotype. *J Photochem Photobiol B* 63: 1-7

[36] Epstein, E. Jr. (2001). Genetic determinants of basal cell carcinoma risk. *Med Pediatr Oncol* 36: 555-558

[37] Madan, V.; Hoban, P.; Strange, R.C.; Fryer, A.A. & Lear, J.T. (2006). Genetics and risk factors for basal cell carcinoma. *Br J Dermatol* 154: 5-7

[38] Roewert-Huber, J.; Lange-Asschenfeldt, B.; Stockfleth, E. & Kerl, H. (2007). Epidemiology and aetiology of basal cell carcinoma. *Brit J Dermatol* 157 (Suppl. 2): 47-51

[39] Dessinioti, C.; Antoniou, C.; Katsambas, A. & Stratigos, A.J. (2010). Basal cell carcinoma: what's new under the sun. *Photochem Photobiol* 86: 481-491

[40] Jones, E.A.; Sajid, M.I.; Shenton, A. & Evans, D.G. (2011). Basal cell carcinomas in gorlin syndrome: a review of 202 patients. *J Skin Cancer,* Volume 2011, Article ID 217378, 6 pages

[41] Parren, L.J. & Frank, J. (2011). Hereditary tumour syndromes featuring basal cell carcinomas. *Br J Dermatol* 165: 30-34

[42] Vlajinac, H.; Adanja, B.; Lazar, Z.; Bogavac, A.; Bjekic, M.; Marinkovic, J. & Kocev, N. (2000). Risk factors for basal cell carcinoma. *Acta Oncol* 39: 611-616

[43] Lock-Andersen, J.; Drzewiecki, K. & Wulf, H. (1999). Eye and hair colour, skin type and constitutive skin pigmentation as risk factors for basal cell carcinoma and cutaneous malignant melanoma. A Danish case-control study. *Acta Derm Venereol* 79: 74-80

[44] de Villiers, E.; Lavergne, D.; McLaren, K. & Benton, E. (1997). Prevailing papillomavirus types in non-melanoma carcinomas of the skin in renal allograft recipients. *Int J Cancer* 73: 356-361

[45] Harwood, C.A. & Proby, C. (2002). Human papillomaviruses and non-melanoma skin cancer. *Curr Opin Infect Dis* 15: 101-114

[46] Stockfleth, E.; Nindl, I.; Sterry, W.; Ulrich, C.; Schmook, T. & Meyer, T. (2004). Human papillomaviruses in transplant-associated skin cancers. *Dermatol Surg* 30: 604-609

[47] Hannuksela-Svahn, A.; Pukkala, E. & Karvonen, J. (1999). Basal cell skin carcinoma and other nonmelanoma skin cancers in Finland from 1956 through 1995. *Arch Dermatol* 135: 781-786

[48] Stern, R.S. (1999). The mysteries of geographic variability in nonmelanoma skin cancer incidence. *Arch Dermatol* 135: 843-844

[49] Staples, M.; Marks, R. & Giles, G. (1998). Trends in the incidence of non-melanocytic skin cancer (NMSC) treated in Australia 1985-1995: are primary prevention programs starting to have an effect? *Int J Cancer* 78: 144-148

[50] Lear, W.; Dahlke, E. & Murray, C.A. (2007). Basal cell carcinoma: review of epidemiology, pathogenesis, and associated risk factors. *J Cutan Med Surg* 11: 19-30

[51] Richmond-Sinclair, N.M.; Pandeya, N.; Ware, R.S.; Neale, R.E.; Williams, G.M.; van der Pols, J.C. & Green, A.C. (2009). Incidence of basal cell carcinoma multiplicity and detailed anatomic distribution: longitudinal study of an Australian population. *J Invest Dermatol* 129: 323-328

[52] Richmond-Sinclair, N.M.; Pandeya, N.; Williams, G.M.; Neale, R.E.; van der Pols, J.C. & Green, A.C. (2010). Clinical signs of photodamage are associated with basal cell carcinoma multiplicity and site: a 16-year longitudinal study. *Int J Cancer* 127: 2622-2629

[53] Flohil, S.C.; de Vries, E.; Neumann, H.A.; Coebergh, J.W. & Nijsten, T. (2011). Incidence, prevalence and future trends of primary basal cell carcinoma in the Netherlands. *Acta Derm Venereol* 91: 24-30

[54] Sander, C.S.; Hamm, F.; Elsner, P. & Thiele, J.J. (2003). Oxidative stress in malignant melanoma and non-melanoma skin cancer. *Br J Dermatol* 148: 913-922

[55] de Gruijl, F.; van Kranen, H. & Mullenders, L. (2001). UV-induced DNA damage, repair, mutations and oncogenic pathways in skin cancer. *J Photochem Photobiol B* 63: 19-27

[56] de Gruijl, F. (2002). Photocarcinogenesis: UVA vs. UVB radiation. *Skin Pharmacol Appl Skin Physiol* 15: 316-320

[57] Burnworth, B.; Arendt, S.; Muffler, S.; Steinkraus, V.; Brocker, E. B.; Birek, C.; Hartschuh, W.; Jauch, A. & Boukamp, P. (2007). The multi-step process of human skin carcinogenesis: A role for p53, cyclin D1, hTERT, p16, and TSP-1. *Eur J Cell Biol* 86: 763-780

[58] Slaughter, D.; Southwick, H. & Smejkal, W. (1953). "Field cancerization" in oral stratified squamous epithelium. *Cancer* 6: 963-968

[59] Mertens, F.; Heim, S.; Mandahl, N.; Johansson, B.; Mertens, O.; Persson, B.; Salemark, L.; Wennerberg, J.; Jonsson, N. & Mitelman, F. (1991) Cytogenetic analysis of 33 basal cell carcinomas. *Cancer Res* 51: 954-957

[60] Kanjilal, S.; Strom, S.S.; Clayman, G.L.; Weber, R.S.; El-Naggar, A.K.; Kapur, V.; Cummings, K.K.; Hill, L.A.; Spitz, M.R.; Kripke, M.L. & Ananthaswamy, N. (1995). p53 mutations in nonmelanoma skin cancer of the head and neck: molecular evidence for field cancerization. *Cancer Res* 55: 3604-3609

[61] Carlson, J.A.; Scott, D.; Wharton, J. & Sell, S. (2001). Incidental histopathologic patterns: Possible evidence of `field cancerization' surrounding skin tumors. *Amer J Dermatopathol* 23: 494-496

[62] Stern, R.; Bolshakov, S.; Nataraj, A. & Ananthaswamy, H. (2002). p53 mutation in nonmelanoma skin cancers occurring in psoralen ultraviolet A-treated patients: Evidence for heterogeneity and field cancerization. *J Invest Dermatol* 119: 522-526

[63] Ulrich, C.; Kanitakis, J.; Stockfleth, E. & Euvrard, S. (2008). Skin cancer in organ transplant recipients--where do we stand today? *Am J Transplant* 8: 2192-2198

[64] Ueda, M.; Ouhtit, A.; Bito, T.; Nakazawa, K.; Lübbe, J.; Ichihashi, M.; Yamasaki, H. & Nakazawa, H. (1997). Evidence for UV-associated activation of telomerase in human skin. *Cancer Res* 57: 370-374

[65] Hollstein, M.; Sidransky, D.; Vogelstein, B. & Harris, C.C. (1991). p53 mutations in human cancers. *Science* 253: 49-53

[66] Lane, D.P. (1992). p53, guardian of the genome. *Nature* 358: 15-16

[67] Haupt, S.; Berger, M.; Goldberg, Z. & Haupt, Y. (2003). Apoptosis - the p53 network. *J Cell Sci* 116: 4077-4085

[68] Wyllie, A.H. (1993). Apotptose (The 1992 Frank Rose Memorial Lecture). *Br J Cancer* 67: 205-208

[69] Cadwell, C. & Zambetti, G.P. (2001). The effects of wild-type p53 tumor suppressor activity and mutant p53 gain-of-function on cell growth. *Gene* 277: 15-30

[70] Shen, Y. & White, E. (2001). p53-dependent apoptosis pathways. Adv Cancer Res 82: 55-84

[71] Fadeel, B. & Orrenius, S. (2005). Apoptosis: a basic biological phenomenon with wide-ranging implications in human disease. *J Intern Med* 258: 479-517

[72] Foijer, F. & te Riele, H. (2006). Check, double check: the G2 barrier to cancer. *Cell Cycle* 5: 831-835

[73] Zilfou, J.T. & Lowe, S.W. (2009). Tumor suppressive functions of p53. *Cold Spring Harb Perspect Biol* 1: 00: a001883

[74] Tapia, N. & Schöler, H.R. (2010). p53 connects tumorigenesis and reprogramming to pluripotency. *J Exp Med* 207: 2045-2048

[75] Sun, W. & Yang, J. (2010). Functional mechanisms for human tumor suppressors. *J Cancer* 1: 136-140

[76] Ryan, K.M. (2011). p53 and autophagy in cancer: guardian of the genome meets guardian of the proteome. *Eur J Cancer* 47: 44-50

[77] Strasser, A.; Harris, A.; Jacks, T. & Cory, S. (1994). DNA damage can induce apoptosis in proliferating lymphoid cells via p53-independent mechanisms inhibitable by bcl-2. *Cell* 79: 329-339

[78] Chiou, S.-K.; Rao, L. & White, E. (1994). Bcl-2 blocks p53-dependent apoptosis. *Mol Cell Biol* 14: 2556-2563

[79] Norris, D.A. (1995). Differential control of cell death in the skin. *Arch Dermatol* 131: 945-948

[80] Delehedde, M.; Cho, S.; Sarkiss, M.; Brisbay, S.; Davies, M.; El-Naggar, A. & McDonnell, T. (1999). Altered expression of bcl-2 family member proteins in nonmelanoma skin cancer. *Cancer* 85: 1514-1422

[81] Ramdial, P.; Madaree, A.; Reddy, R. & Chetty, R. (2000). Bcl-2 protein expression in aggressive and non-aggressive basal cell carcinomas. *J Cutan Pathol* 27: 283-291

[82] Dicker, T.; Siller, G. & Saunders, N. (2002). Molecular and cellular biology of basal cell carcinoma. *Australas J Dermatol* 43: 241-246

[83] Vega-Memije, E.; De Larios, N.; Waxtein, L. & Dominguez-Soto, L. (2000). Cytodiagnosis of cutaneous basal and squamous cell carcinoma. *Int J Dermatol* 39: 116-120

[84] Christensen, E.; Bofin, A.; Gudmundsdóttir, I. & Skogvoll, E. (2008). Cytological diagnosis of basal cell carcinoma and actinic keratosis, using Papanicolaou and May-Grünwald-Giemsa stained cutaneous tissue smear. *Cytopathology* 19: 316-322

[85] Tellechea, O.; Reis, J.; Domingues, J. & Baptista, A. (1993). Monoclonal antibody Ber EP4 distinguishes basal-cell carcinoma from squamous-cell carcinoma of the skin. *Am J Dermatopathol* 15: 452-455

[86] Beer, T.; Shepherd, P. & Theaker, J. (2000). Ber EP4 and epithelial membrane antigen aid distinction of basal cell, squamous cell and basosquamous carcinomas of the skin. *Histopathology* 37: 218-223

[87] Swanson, P.; Fitzpatrick, M.; Ritter, J.; Glusac, E. & Wick, M. (1998). Immunohistologic differential diagnosis of basal cell carcinoma, squamous cell carcinoma, and trichoepithelioma in small cutaneous biopsy specimens. *J Cutan Pathol* 25: 153-159

[88] Tope, W.; Nowfear-Rad, M. & Kist, D. (2000). Ber-Ep4-positive phenotype differentiates actinic keratosis from superficial basal cell carcinoma. *Dermatol Surg* 26: 415-418

[89] Yada, K.; Kashima, K.; Daa, T.; Kitano, S.; Fujiwara, S. & Yokoyama, S. (2004). Expression of CD10 in basal cell carcinoma. *Am J Dermatopathol* 26: 463-471

[90] Aiad, H.A. & Hanout, H.M. (2007). Immunohistochemical Expression of CD10 in Cutaneous Basal and Squamous Cell Carcinomas. *J Egypt Natl Canc Inst* 19: 195-201

[91] Guttinger, M.; Sutti, F.; Barnier, C.; McKay, C. & Berti, E. (1995). Expression of CD44 standard and variant forms in skin tumors. Loss of CD44 correlates with aggressive potential. *Eur J Dermatol* 5: 398-406

[92] Seelentag, W.K.F.; Günthert, U.; Saremaslani, P.; Futo, E.; Pfaltz, M.; Heitz, P.U. & Roth. J. (1996). CD44 standard and variant isoform expression in human epidermal skin tumors is not correlated with tumor aggressiveness but down-regulated during proliferation and tumor de-differentiation. *Int J Cancer (Pred Oncol)* 69: 218-224

[93] Dietrich, A.; Tanczos, E.; Vanscheidt, W.; Schopf, E. & Simon J. (1997). Detection of CD44 splice variants in formalin fixed, paraffin-embedded specimens of human skin cancer. *J Cutan Pathol* 24: 37-42

[94] Seiter, S.; Tilgen, W.; Herrmann, K.; Schadendorf, D.; Patzelt, E.; Möller, P. & Zöller, M. (1996). Expression of CD44 splice variants in human skin and epidermal tumours. *Virchows Arch* 428: 141-149

[95] Simon, J.; Heider, K.-H.; Dietrich, A.; Wuttig, C.; Schöpf, E.; Adolf, G.; Ponta, H. & Herrlich, P. (1996). Expression of CD44 isoforms in human skin cancer. *Eur J Cancer 32A*: 1394-1400

[96] Son, K.D.; Kim, T.J.; Lee, Y.S.; Park, G.S.; Han, K.T.; Lim, J.S. & Kang, C.S. (2008). Comparative analysis of immunohistochemical markers with invasiveness and histologic differentiation in squamous cell carcinoma and basal cell carcinoma of the skin. *J Surg Oncol* 97: 615-620

[97] Al- Sader, M.; Doyle, E.; Kay, E.; Bennett, M.; Walsh, C.; Curran, B.; Milburn, C. & Leader, M. (1996). Proliferation indexes A comparison between cutaneous basal and squamous cell carcinomas. *J Clin Pathol* 49: 549-551

[98] Park, H.R.; Min, S.K.; Cho, H.D.; Kim, K.H.; Shin, H.S. & Park, Y.E. (2004). Expression profiles of p63, p53, survivin, and hTERT in skin tumors. *J Cutan Pathol* 31: 544-549

[99] Bäckvall, H.; Wolf, O.; Hermelin, H.; Weitzberg, E. & Pontén, F. (2004). The density of epidermal p53 clones is higher adjacent to squamous cell carcinoma in comparison with basal cell carcinoma. *Br J Dermatol* 150: 259-266

[100] Chang, C.; Tsai, R.; Chen, G.; Yu, H. & Chai, C. (1998). Expression of bcl-2, p53 and Ki-67 in arsenical skin cancers. *J Cutan Pathol* 25: 457-462

[101] Bolshakov, S.; Walker, C.; Strom, S.; Selvan, M.; Clayman, G.; El-Naggar, A.; Lippman, S.; Kripke, M. & Ananthaswamy, H. (2003). p53 mutations in human aggressive and nonaggressive basal and squamous cell carcinomas. *Clin Cancer Res* 9: 228-234

[102] Fabricius, E.-M.; Gurr, U. & Wildner, G.-P. (2002). Telomerase activity levels in the surgical margin and tumour distant tissue of the squamous cell carcinoma of the head-and-neck. *Anal Cell Pathol* 24: 25-39

[103] Fabricius, E.-M.; Bezeluk, A.; Kruse-Boitschenko, U.; Wildner, G.-P. & Klein, M. (2003). Clinical significance of telomerase activity in basal cell carcinomas and in tumour-free surgical margins. *Int J Oncol* 23: 1389-1399

[104] Fabricius, E.-M. (2006). The role of telomerase for cancerogenesis of basal cell and squamous cell carcinomas. In: Reichrath J (ed.): *Molecular Mechanisms of Basal Cell and Squamous Cell Carinomas*, New York , Landes Bioscience and Springer Science + Bisness Media Inc., pp 115-133, ISBN 0-387-26046-3

[105] Cordell, J.L.; Falini, B.; Erber, W.N.; Ghosh, A.K.; Abdulaziz, Z.; MacDonald, S.; Pulford, K.A F.; Stein, H. & Mason, D.Y. (1984). Immunoenzymatic labeling of monoclonal antibodies using immune complexes of complexes of alkaline phosphatase and monoclonal anti-alkine phosphatase (APAAP Complexes). *J Histochem Cytochem* 32: 219-229

[106] Fabricius, E.-M.; Kruse-Boitschenko, U.; Khoury, R.; Wildner, G.-P.; Raguse, J.-D. & Klein, M. (2009). Immunohistochemical determination of the appropiate anti-hTERT antibodies for in situ detection of telomerase activity in frozen sections of head and neck squamous cell carcinomas and tumor margin tissues. *Int J Oncol* 34: 1257-1279

[107] Fabricius. E.-M.; Kruse-Boitschenko, U.: Khoury, R.; Wildner, G.-P.; Raguse, J.-D.; Klein, M. & Hoffmeister, B. (2009). Localization of telomerase hTERT protein in frozen sections of basal cell carcinomas (BCC) and tumor margin tissues. *Int J Oncol* 35: 1377-1394

[108] Friedman, H.; Williams, T.; Zamora , S. & al Assaad, Z. (1997). Recurrent basal cell carcinoma in margin-positive tumors. *Ann Plast Surg* 38: 232-235

[109] Rippey, J. & Rippey, E. (1997). Characteristics of incompletely excised basal cell carcinomas of the skin. *Med J Aust* 166: 581-583

[110] Robinson, J. & Fisher, S. (2000). Recurrent basal cell carcinoma after incomplete resection. *Arch Dermatol* 136: 1318-1324

[111] Fleischer, A. J.; Feldman. S.; Barlow, J.; Zheng, B.; Hahn, H.; Chuang, T.; Draft, K.; Golitz, L.; Wu, E.; Katz, A.; Maize, J.; Knapp, T. & Leshin, B. (2001). The specialty of the treating physician affects the likelihood of tumor-free resection margins for basal cell carcinoma: results from a multi-institutional retrospective study. *J Am Acad Dermatol* 44: 224-230

[112] Bisson, M.; Dunkin, C.; Suvarna, S. & Griffiths, R. (2002). Do plastic surgeons resect basal cell carcinomas too widely? A prospective study comparing surgical and histological margins. *Brit J Plast Surg* 55: 293-297

[113] Nagore, E.; Grau, C.; Molinero, J. & Fortea, J.M. (2003). Positive margins in basal cell carcinoma: relationship to clinical features and recurrence risk. A retrospective study of 248 patients. *J Eur Acad Dermatol Venereol* 17: 167-170

[114] Gulleth, Y.; Goldberg, N.; Silverman, R.P & Gastman, B.R. (2010). What is the best surgical margin for a basal cell carcinoma: a meta-analysis of the literature. *Plast Reconstr Surg* 126: 1222-1231

[115] Wittekind, Ch.; Meyer, H.J. & Bootz, F. (Eds) (2005). TNM Klassifikation maligner Tumoren. *UICC International Union Against Cancer*. 6. Aufl. Korr. Nachdruck. Hauttumoren. 111-116

[116] Vico, P.; Fourez, T.; Nemec, E.; Andry, G. & Deraemaecker, R. (1995). Aggressive basal cell carcinoma of head and neck areas. *Eur J Surg Oncol* 21: 490-497

[117] Rippey, J. (1998). Why classify basal cell carcinomas? *Histopathology* 32: 393-398

[118] De Rosa, G.; Vetrani, A.; Zeppa, P.; Zabatta, A.; Barra, E.; Gentile, R.; Fulciniti, F.; Troncone, G.; die Benedetto, G. & Palombini, L. (1990). Comparative morphometric analysis of aggressive and ordinary basal cell carcinoma of the skin. *Cancer* 65: 544-549

[119] De Rosa, G.; Staibano, S.; Barra, E.; Zappa, P.; Salvatore, G.; Vetrani, A. & Palombini, L. (1992). Nucleolar organizer regions in aggressive and nonaggressive basal cell carcinoma of the skin. *Cancer* 69: 123-126

[120] Raasch, B.A.; Buettner, P.G. & Garbe, C. (2006). Basal cell carcinoma: histological classification and body-site distribution. *Br J Dermatol* 155: 401-407

[121] Ansarin, H.; Daliri, M. & Soltani-Arabshahi, R. (2006). Expression of p53 in aggressive and non-aggressive histologic variants of basal cell carcinoma. *Eur J Dermatol* 16: 543-547

[122] Staibano, S.; Lo Muzio, L.; Pannone, G.S.M.; Salvatore, G.; Errico, M.; Fanali, S.; De Rosa, G. & Piattelli, A. (2001). Interaction between bcl-2 and p53 in neoplastic progression in basal cell carcinoma of the head and neck. *Anticancer Res* 21: 3757-3764

[123] Staibano, S.; Lo Muzio, L.; Pannone, G.; Somma, P.; Farronato, G.; Franco, R.; Bambini, F.; Serpico, R. & De Rosa, G. (2001). P53 and hMSH2 expression in basal cell carcinomas and malignant melanomas from photoexposed areas of head and neck region. *Int J Oncol* 19: 551-559

[124] Staibano, S.; Lo Muzio, L.; Mezza, E.; Argenziano, G.; Tornillo, L.; Pannone, G. & De Rosa, G. (1999). Prognostic value of apoptotic index in cutaneous basal cell carcinomas of head and neck. *Oral Oncol* 35: 541-547

[125] Staibano, S.; Lo Muzio, L.; Pannone, G.; Mezza, E.; Argenziano, G.; Vetrani, A.; Lucariello, A.; Franco, R.; Errico, M. & DeRosa, G. (2001). DNA ploidy and cyclin D1 expression in basal cell carcinoma of the head and neck. *Am J Clin Pathol* 115: 805-813

[126] Staibano, S.; Boscaino, A.; Salvatore, G.; Orabona, P.; Palombini, L. & De Rosa, G. (1996). The prognostic significance of tumor angiogenesis in nonaggressive and aggressive basal cell carcinoma of the human skin. *Hum Pathol* 27: 695-700

[127] Günthert, U. (1993). CD44: A multitude of isoforms with diverse functions. *Curr Top Microbiol Immunol* 184: 47-63

[128] Naor, D.; Sionov, R. & Ish-Shalom, D. (1997). CD44: Structure, function, and association with the malignant process. *Adv Cancer Res* 71: 241-319

[129] Naor, D.; Sionov, R.V. & Ish-Shalom, D. (2002). CD44 in cancer. *Crit Rev Clin Lab Sci* 39: 527-579

[130] Hyckel, P.; Kosmehl, H.; Berndt, A.; Hesse, J.; Stiller, K.J. & Robotta, C. (1995). Immunohistochemische Demonstration von CD 44 H, CD 44 v3 und CD 44 v6 im oralen Plattenepithelkarzinom. Dtsch Z Mund Kiefer GesichtsChir 19: 284-289

[131] Fabricius, E.-M.; Langford, A.; Bier, J.; Hell, B.; Wildner, G.-P. & Blümcke, S. (1997). Immunohistochemical characterization of E48 and CD44-v6 expression in head and neck carcinomas. *Cancer J* 10: 325-330

[132] Fabricius, E.-M.; Guschmann, M.; Wildner, G.-P.; Langford, A.; Hell, B. & Bier J. (1998). Divergent immunohistochemical E48 and CD44-v6 antigen expression patterns between lymph node metastases and primary squamous cell carcinomas in the head and neck region. *Cancer J* 11: 325-330

[133] Fabricius, E.-M.; Guschmann, M.; Langford, A.; Hell, B. & Bier, J. (2000). Immunohistochemical assessment of the tumour-associated epitopes CD44v6 and E48 in tumour-free lymph nodes from patients with squamous cell carcinoma in the head-neck region. *Anal Cell Pathol* 20: 115-129

[134] Salmi, M.; Grön-Virta, K.; Sointu, P.; Grenman, R.; Kalimo, H. & Jalkanen, S. (1993). Regulated expression of exon v6 containing isoforms of CD44 in man: downregulation during malignant tranformation of tumors of squamocellular origin. *J Cell Biol* 122: 431-442

[135] Baum, H.P.; Schmid, T.; Shock, G. & Reichrath, J. (1996). Expression of CD44 isoforms in basal cell carcinomas. *Br J Dermatol* 134: 465-468

[136] Kooy, A.; Tank, B.; de Jong, A.; Vuzevski, V.; van der Kwast, T. & van Joost, T. (1999). Expression of E-cadherin, alpha- & beta-catenin, and CD44V6 and the subcellular localization of E-cadherin and CD44V6 in normal epidermis and basal cell carcinoma. *Hum Pathol* 30: 1328-1335

[137] Dingemans, K.; Ramkema, M.; Koopman, G.; Van Der Wal, A.; Das, P. & Pals, S. (1999). The expression of CD44 glycoprotein adhesion molecules in basal cell carcinomas is related to growth pattern and invasiveness. *Br J Dermatol* 140: 17-25

[138] Dingemans, K.; Ramkema, M. & Pals, S. (2002). CD44 is exposed to the extracellular matrix at invasive sites in basal cell carcinomas. *Lab Invest* 82: 313-322

[139] Schrijvers, A.H.G.J.; Gerretsen, M.; Fritz, J.M. ; van Walsum, M.; Quak, J. J.; Snow, G.B. & van Dongen, G.A.M. S. (1991). Evidence for a role of the monoclonal antibody E48 defined antigen in cell-cell adhesion in squamous epithelia and head and neck squamous cell carcinoma. *Exper Cell Res* 196: 264-269

[140] Quak, J.J.; Balm, A.J.M.; van Dongen, G .A.M. S.; Brakkee, J.G.P.; Scheper, R. J.; Snow, G.B. & Meijer, C. J.M. (1990). A 22-kd surface antigen detected by monoclonal antibody E 48 is exlusively expressed in stratified squamous and transitional epithelia. *Am J Pathol* 136: 191-197

[141] Schrijvers, A.H.; Quak, J.J.; Uyterlinde, A.M.; van Walsum, M.; Meijer, C.J.; Snow, G.B. & van Dongen, G.A. (1993). MAb U36, a novel monoclonal antibody successful in

immunotargeting of squamous cell carcinoma of the head and neck. *Cancer Res* 53: 4383-4390

[142] van Hal, N.L.W.; van Dongen, G.A.M.S.; Rood-Knippels, E.M.C.; van Valk, P.; Snow, G.B. & Brakenhoff, R.H. (1996). Monoclonal antibody U36, a suitable candidate for clinical immunotherapy of squamous-cell carcinoma, recognizes a CD44 isoform. *Int J Cancer* 68: 520-527

[143] Van Hal, N.; van Dongen, G.; TenBrink, C.; Herron, J.; Snow, G. & Brakenhoff, R. (1997). Sequence variation in the monoclonal-antibody-U36-defined CD44v6 epitope. *Cancer Immunol Immunother* 45: 88-92

[144] Remmele, W.; Hildebrand, U.; Hienz, H.A.; Klein, P.-J.; Vierbuchen, M.; Behnken, L.J.; Heicke, B. & Scheidt, E. (1986). Comparative histological, histochemical, immunohistochemical and biochemical studies on oestrogen receptors, lectin receptors, and Barr bodies in human breast cancer. *Virchows Arch (Pathol Anat)* 409: 127-147

[145] Remmele, W. & Stegner, H.E. (1987). Vorschlag zur einheitlichen Definition eines immunreaktiven Scores (IRE) für den immunhistochemischen Östrogenrezeptor-Nachweis (ER-ICA) im Mammagewebe. *Pathologie* 8: 138-140

[146] de Bree, R.; Ross, J.; Quak, J.; den Hollander, W.; Snow, G. & van Dongen, G. (1995). Radioimmunoscintigraphy and biodistribution of technetium-99m-labeled monoclonal antibody U36 in patient with head and neck cancer. *Clin Cancer Res* 1: 591-598

[147] Börjesson, P.K.; Postema, E.J.; de Bree, R.; Roos, J.C.; Leemans, C.R.; Kairemo, K.J. & van Dongen, G.A. (2004). Radioimmunodetection and radioimmunotherapy of head and neck cancer. *Oral Oncol* 40: 761-772

[148] Colnot, D.R.; Nieuwenhuis, E.J.; Kuik, D.J.; Leemans, C.R.; Dijkstra, J.; Snow, G.B.; van Dongen, G.A. & Brakenhoff, R.H. (2004). Clinical significance of micrometastatic cells detected by E48 (Ly-6D) reverse transcription-polymerase chain reaction in bone marrow of head and neck cancer patients. *Clin Cancer Res* 10: 7827-7833

[149] Börjesson, P.K.; Jauw, Y.W.; Boellaard, R.; de Bree, R.; Comans, E.F.; Roos, J.C.; Castelijns, J.A.; Vosjan, M.J.; Kummer, J.A.; Leemans, C.R.; Lammertsma, A.A. & van Dongen, G.A. (2006). Performance of immuno-positron emission tomography with zirconium-89-labeled chimeric monoclonal antibody U36 in the detection of lymph node metastases in head and neck cancer patients. *Clin Cancer Res* 12: 2133-2140

[150] Fortin, M.A.; Salnikov, A.V.; Nestor, M.; Heldin, N.E.; Rubin, K. & Lundqvist, H. (2007). Immuno-PET of undifferentiated thyroid carcinoma with radioiodine-labelled antibody cMAb U36: application to antibody tumour uptake studies. *Eur J Nucl Med Mol Imaging* 34: 1376-1387

[151] Sandström, K.; Nestor, M.; Ekberg, T.; Engström, M.; Anniko, M. & Lundqvist, H. (2008). Targeting CD44v6 expressed in head and neck squamous cell carcinoma: preclinical characterization of an ^{111}In-labeled monoclonal antibody. *Tumour Biol* 29: 137-144

[152] Börjesson, P.K.; Jauw, Y.W.; de Bree, R.; Roos, J.C.; Castelijns, J.A.; Leemans, C.R.; van Dongen, G.A. & Boellaard, R.(2009). Radiation dosimetry of ^{89}Zr-labeled chimeric monoclonal antibody U36 as used for immuno-PET in head and neck cancer patients. *J Nucl Med* 50: 1828-1836

[153] de Bree, R.; Roos, J.; Plaizier, M.; Quak, J.; van Kamp, G.; den Hollander, W.; Snow, G. & van Dongen, G. (1997). Selection of monoclonal antibody E48 IgG or U36 IgG for adjuvant radioimmunotherapy in head and neck cancer patients. *Brit J Cancer* 75: 1049-1060

[154] Colnot, D.R.; Quak, J.J.; Roos, J.C.; van Lingen, A.; Wilhelm, A.J.; van Kamp, G.J.; Huijgens, P.C.; Snow, G.B. & van Dongen, G.A. (2000). Phase I therapy study of ^{186}Re-labeled chimeric monoclonal antibody U36 in patients with squamous cell carcinoma of the head and neck. *J Nucl Med* 41: 1999-2010

[155] Börjesson, P.K.; Postema, E.J.; Roos, J.C.; Colnot, D.R.; Marres, H.A.; van Schie, M.H.; Stehle, G.; de Bree, R.; Snow, G.B.; Oyen, W.J. & van Dongen, G.A. (2003). Phase I therapy study with (186)Re-labeled humanized monoclonal antibody BIWA 4 (bivatuzumab) in patients with head and neck squamous cell carcinoma. *Clin Cancer Res* 9: 3961S- 3972S

[156] Colnot, D.R.; Roos, J.C.; de Bree, R.; Wilhelm, A.J.; Kummer, J.A.; Hanft, G.; Heider, K.H.; Stehle, G.; Snow, G.B.; & van Dongen, G.A. (2003). Safety, biodistribution, pharmacokinetics, and immunogenicity of ^{99m}Tc-labeled humanized monoclonal antibody BIWA 4 (bivatuzumab) in patients with squamous cell carcinoma of the head and neck. *Cancer Immunol Immunother* 52: 576-582

[157] Urano, Y.; Assano, T.; Yoshimoto, K.; Iwahana, H.; Kubu, Y.; Kato, S.; Sasaki, S.; Takeuchi, N.; Uchida, N.; Nakanishi, H.; Arase, S. & Itakura, M. (1995). Frequent p53 accumulation in the chronically sun-exposed epidermis and clonal expansion of p53 mutant cells in the epidermis adjacent to basal cell carcinoma. *J Invest Dermatol* 104: 928-932

[158] Barrett, T.L.; Smith, K.J.; Hodge, J.J.; Butler, R.; Hall, F.W. & Skelton, H.G. (1997). Immunohistochemical nuclear staining for p53, PCNA, and Ki-67 in different histologic variants of basal cell carcinoma. *J Am Acad Dermatol* 37: 430-437

[159] Demirkan, N.; Colakoglu, N. & Duzcan, E. (2000). Value of p53 protein in biological behavior of basal cell carcinoma and in normal epithelia adjacent to carcinomas. *Pathol Oncol Res* 6: 272-274

[160] Rajabi, M.A.; Rajabi, P. & Afshar-Moghaddam, N. (2006). Determination of p53 expression in basal cell carcinoma tissues and adjacent nontumoral epidermis from sun-exposed areas of the head and neck. *Arch Iran Med* 9: 46-48

[161] Koseoglu, R.D.; Sezer, E.; Eyibilen, A.; Aladag, I. & Etikan, I. (2009). Expressions of p53, cyclinD1 and histopathological features in basal cell carcinomas. *J Cutan Pathol* 36: 958-965

[162] Fabricius, E.-M.; Kruse-Boitschenko, U.; Schneeweiss, U.; Wildner, G.-P; Hoffmeister, B. & Raguse, J.-D. (2011). Model examination of chemoprevention with retinoids in squamous cell carcinomas of the head and neck region and suitable biomarkers for chemoprevention. *Int J Oncol* 39: 1083-1097

[163] Healy, E.; Angus, B.; Lawrence, C.M. & Rees, J.L. (1995). Prognostic value of Ki67 antigen expression in basal cell carcinomas. *Br J Dermatol* 133: 737-741

[164] Abdelsayed, R.A.; Guijarro-Rojas, M.; Ibrahim, N.A. & Sangueza, O.P. (2000). Immunohistochemical evaluation of basal cell carcinoma and trichepithelioma using bcl-2, Ki67, PCNA and p53. *J Cutan Pathol* 27: 169-175

[165] Greider, C. & Blackburn, E. (1987). The telomere terminal transferase of Tetrahymena is a ribonucleoprotein enzyme with two kinds of primer specificity. *Cell* 51: 887-898

[166] Greider, C. & Blackburn, E. (1995). Identification of a specific telomere terminal transferase activity in Tetrahymena extracts. *Cell* 43: 405-413
[167] Hayflick, L. & Moorhead, P. (1961). The serial cultivation of human diploid cell strains. *Exper Cell Res* 25: 585-624
[168] Kim, N.W.; Piatyszek, M.A.; Prowse, K.R.;, Harley, C.B.; West, M.D.; Ho, P.L.C.; Coviello, G.M.; Wright, W.E.; Weinrich, S.L. & Shay, J.W. (1994) Specific association of human telomerase activity with immortal cells and cancer. *Science* 266: 2011-2015
[169] Wright, W.; Piatyszek, M.R.W.; Byrd, W. & Shay, J. (1996). Telomerase activity in human germline and embryonic tissues and cells. *Dev Genet* 18: 173-179
[170] Hiyama, K.; Hirai, Y.; Kyoizumi, S.; Akiyama, M.; Hiyama, E.; Piatyszek, M.-A.; Shay, J.-W.; Ishioka, S. & Yamakido, M. (1995). Activation of telomerase in human lymphocytes and hematopoietic progenitor cells. *J Immunol* 155: 3711-3715
[171] McKenzie, K.; Umbricht, C. & Sukumar, S. (1999). Applications of telomerase research in the fight against cancer. *Mol Med Today* 5: 114-122
[172] Meyerson, M. (2000). Role of telomerase in normal and cancer cells. *J Clin Oncol* 18: 2626-2634
[173] Ramirez, R.; Wright, W.; Shay, J. & Taylor, R. (1997). Telomerase activity concentrates in the mitotically active segments of human hair follicles. *J Invest Dermatol* 108: 113-117
[174] Matthews, P. & Jones, C. (2001). Clinical implications of telomerase detection. *Histopathology* 38: 485-498
[175] Hoogduijn, M.J.; Gorjup, E. & Genever, P.G. (2006). Comparative characterization of hair follicle dermal stem cells and bone marrow mesenchymal stem cells. *Stem Cells Dev* 15: 49-60
[176] Bodnar, A.; Kim, N.; Effros, R. & Chiu, C.-P. (1996). Mechanism of telomerase induction during T cell activation. *Exp Cell Res* 228: 58-64
[177] Mimeault, M. & Batra, S.K. (2010). Recent advances on skin-resident stem/progenitor cell functions in skin regeneration, aging and cancers and novel anti-aging and cancer therapies. *J Cell Mol Med* 14: 116-134
[178] Effros, R.B. (2011). Telomere/telomerase dynamics within the human immune system: effect of chronic infection and stress. *Exp Gerontol* 46: 135-140
[179] de Lange, T. (1994). Activation of telomerase in a human tumor. Proc Natl Acad Sci USA 91: 2882-2885
[180] Shay, J. & Wright, W. (1996). The reactivation of telomerase activity in cancer progression. *Trends Genetic* 12: 129-131
[181] Shay, J. & Bacchetti, S. (1997). A survey of telomerase activity in human cancer. *Eur J Cancer* 33: 787-791
[182] Dhaene, K.; van Marck, E. & Parwaresch, R. (2000). Telomeres, telomerase and cancer: an up-date. Virchows Arch 437: 1-16
[183] Taylor, R.; Ramirez, R.; Ogoshi, M.; Chaffins, M.; Piatyszek, M. & Shay, J. (1996). Detection of telomerase activity in malignant and nonmalignant skin conditions. *J Invest Dermatol* 106: 759-765
[184] Parris, C.; Jezzard, S.; Silver, A.; MacKie, R.; McGregor, J. & Newbold, R. (1999). Telomerase activity in melanoma and non-melanoma skin cancer. *Br J Cancer* 79: 47-53
[185] Wu, A.; Ichihashi, M. & Ueda, M. (1999). Correlation of the expression of human telomerase subunits with telomerase activity in normal skin and skin tumors. *Cancer* 86: 2038-2044

[186] Kim, B.-C.; Ryoo, Y.-W. &, Lee, K.-S. (2000). Telomerase activity in squamous cell carcinoma and basal cell carcinoma. *Korean J Invest Dermatol* 7: 184-187

[187] Chen, Z.; Smith, K.; Skelton, H.; Barrett, T.; Greenway, H.J. &, Lo, S. (2001). Telomerase activity in Kaposi's sarcoma, squamous cell carcinoma, and basal cell carcinoma. *Exp Biol Med (Maywood)* 226: 753-757

[188] Boldrini, L.; Loggini, B.; Gisfredi, S.; Zucconi, Y.; Di Quirico, D.; Biondi, R.; Cervadoro, G.; Barachini, P.; Basolo, F.; Pingitore, R. & Fontanini, G. (2003). Evaluation of telomerase in non-melanoma skin cancer. *Int J Mol Med* 11: 607-611

[189] Saleh, S.; King-Yin Lam, A.; Buettner, P.G.; Glasby, M.; Raasch, B. & Ho, Y.H. (2007). Telomerase activity of basal cell carcinoma in patients living in North Queensland, Australia. *Hum Pathol* 38: 1023-1029

[190] Nakamura, T.M.; Morin, G.B.; Chapman, K.B. ; Weinrich, S.L.; Andrews,W.H.R.; Lingner, J.; Harley, C.B. & Cech, T. (1997). Telomerase catalytic subunit homologs from fission yeast and human. *Science* 277: 955-959

[191] Harrington, L.; Zhou, W.; McPhail, T.; Oulton, R.; Yeung, D.; Mar, Y.; Bass, M. & Robinson, M. (1997). Human telomerase contains evolutionarily conserved catalytic and structural subunits. *Genes Dev* 11: 3109-3115

[192] Hu, S.; Chan, H.L.; Chen, M.C. & Pang, J.H. (2002). Telomerase expression in benign and malignant skin neoplasms: comparison of three major subunits. *J Formos Med Assoc* 101: 593-597

[193] Ogoshi, M.; Le, T.; Shay, J. & Taylor, R. (1998). In situ hybridization analysis of the expression of human telomerase RNA in normal and pathologic conditions of the skin. *J Invest Dermatol* 110: 818-823

[194] Attia, E.A.; Seada, L.S.; El-Sayed, M.H. & El-Shiemy, S.M. (2010). Study of telomerase reverse transcriptase (hTERT) expression in normal, aged, and photo-aged skin. *Int J Dermatol* 49: 886-893

[195] Wu, Y.L.; Dudognon, C.; Nguyen, E.; Hillion, J.; Pendino, F.; Tarkanyi, I.; Aradi, J.; Lanotte, M.; Tong, J.H.; Chen, G.Q. & Segal-Bendirdjian, E. (2006). Immunodetection of human telomerase reverse-transcriptase (hTERT) re-appraised: nucleolin and telomerase cross paths. *J Cell Sci* 119: 2797-2806

[196] Kyo, S.; Masutomi, K.; Maida, Y.; Kanaya, T.; Yatabe, N.; Nakamura, M., Tanaka, M.; Takarada, M.; Sugawara, I.; Murakami, S.; Taira, T. &, Inoue, M. (2003). Significance of immunological detection of human telomerase reverse transcriptase: re-evaluation of expression and localization of human telomerase reverse transcriptase. *Am J Pathol* 163: 859-867

[197] Sun, P.M.; Wei, L.H.; Luo, M.Y.; Liu, G.; Wang, J.L.; Mustea, A.; Könsgen, D.; Lichtenegger, W. & Sehouli, J. (2007). The telomerase activity and expression of hTERT gene can serve as indicators in the anti-cancer treatment of human ovarian cancer. *Eur J Obstet Gynecol Reprod Biol* 130: 149-157

[198] Ulrich, C.; Jürgensen, J.S.; Degen, A.; Hackethal, M.; Ulrich, M.; Patel, M.J.; Eberle, J.; Terhorst, D.; Sterry, W. & Stockfleth, E. (2009). Prevention of non-melanoma skin cancer in organ transplant patients by regular use of a sunscreen: a 24 months, prospective, case-control study. *Br J Dermatol* 161 (Suppl. 3): 78-84

[199] Einspahr, J.G.; Bowden, G.T. & Alberts, D.S. (2003). Skin cancer chemoprevention: strategies to save our skin. *Recent Results Cancer Res* 163: 151-164, discussion 264-266

[200] Peck, G.L.; DiGiovanna, J.J.; Sarnoff, D.S.; Gross, E.G.; Butkus, D.; Olsen, T.G. & Yoder, F.W. (1988). Treatment and prevention of basal cell carcinoma with oral isotretinoin. *J Am Acad Dermatol* 19: 176-185

[201] Greenberg, E.R.; Baron, J.A.;, Stukel, T.A.; Stevens, M.M.; Mandel, J.S.; Spencer, S.K.; Elias, P.M.; Lowe, N.; Nierenberg, D.W.; Bayrd, G.; Vance, J.C.; Freeman, D.H. Jr.; Clendenning, W.E.; Kwan, T. & the Skin Cancer Prevention Study Group (1990). A clinical trial of beta carotene to prevent basal-cell and squamous-cell cancers of the skin. *N Engl J Med* 323: 789-795

[202] Tangrea, J.A.; Edwards, B.K.; Taylor, P.R.; Hartman, A.M.; Peck, G.L.; Salasche, S.J.; Menon, P.A.; Benson, P.M.; Mellette, J.R.; Guill, M.A.;Robinson, J.K.; Gui, J.D.; Stoll,H.L.; Grabski, W.J.; Winton, G.B. & other members of the Isotretinoin-Basal Cell Carcinoma Study Group (1992). Long-term therapy with low-dose isotretinoin for prevention of basal cell carcinoma: a multicenter clinical trial. Isotretinoin-Basal Cell Carcinoma Study Group. *J Natl Cancer Inst* 84: 328-332

[203] Levine, N.; Moon, T.E.; Cartmel, B.; Bangert, J.L.; Rodney, S.; Dong, Q.; Peng, Y.M. & Alberts, D.S. (1997). Trial of retinol and isotretinoin in skin cancer prevention: a randomized, double-blind, controlled trial. Southwest Skin Cancer Prevention Study Group. *Cancer Epidemiol Biomarkers Prev* 6: 957-961

[204] Tsao, A.S.; Kim, E.S. & Hong, W.K. (2004). Chemoprevention of cancer. *CA Cancer J Clin* 54: 150-180

[205] Otley, C.C.; Stasko, T.; Tope, W.D. & Lebwo, M. (2006). Chemoprevention of nonmelanoma skin cancer with systemic retinoids: practical dosing and management of adverse effects. *Dermatol Surg* 32: 562-568

[206] Campbell, R.M. & DiGiovanna, J.J. (2006). Skin cancer chemoprevention with systemic retinoids: an adjunct in the management of selected high-risk patients. *Dermatol Ther* 19: 306-314

[207] Clouser, M.C.; Roe, D.J.; Foote, J.A.; Harris, R.B. & Alberts, D.S. (2010). Dose response of retinol and isotretinoin in the prevention of nonmelanoma skin cancer recurrence. *Nutr Cancer* 62: 1058-1066

[208] Lindelöf, B.; Sigurgeirsson, B.; Gäbel, H. & Stern, R. (2000). Incidence of skin cancer in 5356 patients following organ transplantation. *Br J Dermatol* 143: 513-519

[209] Ulrich, C.; Schmook, T.; Sachse, M.M.; Sterry, W. & Stockfleth, E. (2004). Comparative epidemiology and pathogenic factors for nonmelanoma skin cancer in organ transplant patients. *Dermatol Surg* 30: 622-627

[210] De Graaf, Y.G.; Euvrard, S. & Bouwes Bavinck, J.N. (2004). Systemic and topical retinoids in the management of skin cancer in organ transplant recipients. *Dermatol Surg* 30: 656-661

[211] Lippman, S.M.; Heyman, R.A.; Kurie, J.M.; Benner, S.E. & Hong, W.K. (1995): Retinoids and chemoprevention: clinical and basic studies. *J Cell Biochem* 22: 1-10

[212] Chandraratna, R.A. (1996). Tazarotene—first of a new generation of receptor-selective retinoids. *Br J Dermatol* 135: 18-25

[213] Kelloff, G.J. (2000). Perspectives on cancer chemoprevention research and drug development. *Adv Cancer Res* 78: 199-334

[214] Sun, S.Y. & Lotan, R. (2002). Retinoids and their receptors in cancer development and chemoprevention. *Crit Rev Oncol Hematol* 41: 41-55

[215] Dawson, M.I. & Zhang, X.K. (2002). Discovery and design of retinoic acid receptor and retinoid X receptor class- and subtype-selective synthetic analogs of all-trans-retinoic acid and 9-cis-retinoic acid. *Curr Med Chem* 9: 623-637

[216] Dawson, M.I. (2004). Synthetic retinoids and their nuclear receptors. *Curr Med Chem Anticancer Agents* 4: 199-230

[217] Bianchi, L.; Orlandi, A.; Campione, E.; Angeloni, C.; Costanzo, A.; Spagnoli, L.G. & Chimenti, S. (2004). Topical treatment of basal cell carcinoma with tazarotene: a clinicopathological study on a large series of cases. *Br J Dermatol* 151: 148-156

[218] Mangelsdorf, D.J.; Ong, E.S.; Dyck, J.A. & Evans, R.M. (1990). Nuclear receptor that identifies a novel retinoic acid response pathway. *Nature* 345: 224-228

[219] Heyman, R.A.; Mangelsdorf, D.J.; Dyck, J.A.; Stein, R.B.; Eichele, G.; Evans, R.M. & Thaller, C. (1992). 9-cis retinoic acid is a high affinity ligand for the retinoid X receptor. *Cell* 68: 397-406

[220] So, P.L.; Fujimoto, M.A. & Epstein, E.H. Jr. (2008). Pharmacologic retinoid signaling and physiologic retinoic acid receptor signaling inhibit basal cell carcinoma tumorigenesis. *Mol Cancer Ther* 7: 1275-1284

[221] Einspahr, J.; Alberts, D.; Aickin, M.; Welch, K.; Bozzo, P.; Levine, N. & Grogan, T. (1996). Evaluation of proliferating cell nuclear antigen as a surrogate end point biomarker in actinic keratosis and adjacent, normal-appearing, and non-sun-exposed human skin samples. *Cancer Epidemiol Biomarkers Prev* 5: 343-348

[222] Einspahr, J.; Alberts, D.; Aickin, M.; Welch, K.; Bozzo, P.; Grogan, T. & Nelson, M. (1997). Expression of p53 protein in actinic keratosis, adjacent, normal-appearing, and non-sun-exposed human skin. *Cancer Epidemiol Biomarkers Prev* 6: 583-587

[223] Kelloff, G.J.; Sigman, C.C.; Johnson, K.M.; Boone, C.W.; Greenwald, P.; Crowell, J.A.; Hawk, E.T. & Doody, L.A. (2000). Perspectives on surrogate end points in the development of drugs that reduce the risk of cancer. *Cancer Epidemiol Biomarkers Prev* 9: 127-137

[224] Einspahr, J.G.; Stratton, S.P.; Bowden, G.T. & Alberts, D.S. (2002). Chemoprevention of human skin cancer. *Crit Rev Oncol Hematol* 41: 269-285

[225] Orlandi, A.; Bianchi, L.; Costanzo, A.; Campione, E.; Spagnoli, L.G. & Chimenti, S. (2004). Evidence of increased apoptosis and reduced proliferation in basal cell carcinomas treated with tazarotene. *J Invest Dermatol* 122: 1037-1041

[226] Kamradt, J. & Reichrath, J. (1996). Expression of retinoic acid receptor proteins in basal cell carcinomas: an immunohistochemical analysis. *J Histochem Cytochem* 44: 1415-1420

[227] Hartmann, F.; Kosmidis, M.; Mühleisen, B.; French, L.E. & Hofbauer, G.F. (2010). Retinoic acid receptor isoform mRNA expression differs between BCC and SCC of the skin. *Arch Dermatol* 146: 675-676

[228] Reichrath,J; Mittmann, M.; Kamradt, J. & Müller, S.M. (1997). Expression of retinoid-X receptors (-alpha,-beta,-gamma) and retinoic acid receptors (-alpha,-beta,-gamma) in normal human skin: an immunohistological evaluation. *Histochem J* 29: 127-133

[229] Leung, K. (2007). ^{124}I-Anti-CD44v6 chimeric monoclonal antibody U36. Molecular Imaging and Contrast Agent Database (MICAD) [Internet] Bethesda (MD). *National Center for Biotechnology Information (US)*: 1-3

[230] Leung, K. (2010). ^{89}Zr-N-Succinyldesferal-anti-CD44v6 chimeric monoclonal antibody U36. Molecular Imaging and Contrast Agent Database (MICAD) [Internet] Bethesda (MD). *National Center for Biotechnology Information (US)*: 1-3

3

BCC and the Secret Lives of Patched: Insights from Patched Mouse Models

Zhu Juan Li and Chi-chung Hui
Program in Developmental and Stem Cell Biology, Hospital for Sick Children and Department of Molecular Genetics, University of Toronto Canada

1. Introduction

The Hedgehog (Hh) signaling pathway is critical for growth control and patterning during embryonic development and adult homeostasis (Jiang and Hui 2008). The identification of loss-of-function mutations in *PATCHED1* (*PTCH1*) as the underlying cause of nevoid basal cell carcinoma syndrome (Gorlin 2004), which predisposes patients to the development of neoplasms including basal cell carcinoma (BCC), first implicated the involvement of the Hh pathway in tumorigenesis (Johnson et al., 1996; Hahn et al., 1996). PTCH1 is a Hh-binding membrane receptor and functions as a major negative regulator of the pathway by inhibiting the signaling membrane protein SMOOTHENED (SMO). Inactivating mutations in PTCH1 as well as activating mutations in SMO are commonly found in BCC, and it is well established that abnormal Hh pathway activation is the underlying cause of BCC (Reifenberger et al., 2005; Ruiz i Altaba, 2006). However, how pathway activation disrupts normal skin homeostasis to promote BCC formation remains poorly understood.

This chapter provides an overview of the Hh pathway and the role of Ptc receptors during normal skin homeostasis and tumorigenesis. The Patched mouse model provides an excellent tool to study BCC pathogenesis since these mice recapitulate many clinical features of human BCC. In addition, the mouse Ptc1 protein is 95% identical to its human counterpart PTCH1. Examples of how Patched mouse models have facilitated our understanding of the molecular genetic and cellular events of BCC biology will be discussed. In particular, we will focus on studies performed to tease out the biological function of the C-terminal domain of Ptc and its role not only in tumorigenesis but also stem cell biology and cell cycle progression.

2. Patched: The link between BCC and Hh signaling

BCC typically arises in sun-exposed skin and is the most commonly diagnosed cancer in the Caucasian population, with over one million people diagnosed every year in the United States. Despite the high incidence, mortality rate is low, as BCCs rarely metastasize and are generally locally invasive. The vast majority of BCCs arise sporadically, although some are attributed to a genetic predisposition syndrome. NBCCS (Nevoid basal cell carcinoma syndrome, also known as Basal-cell syndrome or Gorlin syndrome, OMIM#109400) is a rare autosomal dominant disease in which individuals display a spectrum of developmental disorders including skeletal malformations, neural tube closure defects, and general overgrowth of the body (Gorlin 2004, Gorlin and Goltz 1960). These patients are highly susceptible to medulloblastoma (MB) of the cerebellum, rhabdomyosarcoma (RMS) of the soft tissue and more frequently BCC.

A link between BCC and the Hh signaling pathway was discovered in 1996, when two independent groups used positional cloning to identify germline mutations in *PTCH1* (9q22.3) in patients with NBCCS and sporadic BCC (Johnson et al., 1996; Hahn et al., 1996). This discovery was seminal in understanding the genetic underpinnings of BCC and aided researchers in developing a suitable animal model. Transgenic mice that overexpress Sonic hedgehog (SHH), the ligand for PTCH1, in the skin develop many features of NBCCS including BCC (Oro et al., 1997). In subsequent years, activating mutations in SMO were reported in patients with sporadic BCC (Xie et al., 1998). These studies highlight the importance and close connection between Hh signaling and BCC biology.

2.1 Hh signaling in the skin

Vertebrate Hh signal transduction occurs in the primary cilium, a microtubule-rich organelle that protrudes from the cell surface of virtually all mammalian cells (reviewed in Goetz and Anderson 2010). Many key components of the Hh pathway are localized to the cilium and, in response to Hh stimulus, they dynamically shuttle in or out of this organelle (May et al., 2005). In vertebrates, there are three Hh ligands: Sonic hedgehog (Shh), Dessert Hh (Dhh) and Indian Hh (Ihh). While *Shh* is more broadly expressed in tissues, including the skin, neural tube and the limb, the action and expression of other ligands are more restricted: *Dhh* in the testis and *Ihh* in the bone. In the absence of the Hh ligand, Ptc is found at the base of the primary cilium and it acts to inhibit the activity of an obligatory transmembrane protein Smo, which normally resides in intracellular vesicles (Figure 1). The binding of Hh to Ptc promotes its migration out of the cilium, allowing the activation and translocation of Smo to the tip. Though the mechanism is unclear, Smo signals downstream to generate activator forms of Gli transcription factors that turn on the expression of Hh-target genes, such as *Ptc1* and *Gli1* (Figure 1). Mutation in components of the intraflagellar transport (IFT) machinery, which is required for cilia production and maintenance, leads to patterning defects in Hh-dependent tissues such as the neural tube and the limb (Huangfu and Anderson 2005; Liu et al., 2005). Depending on the tissue, loss of IFT function during embryogenesis can result in low or high Hh activity as IFTs are required to generate both activator and repressor forms of Gli transcription factors (Huangfu and Anderson 2005; Liu et al., 2005; May et al., 2005). The dual function of cilia on Hh signaling is also revealed in adult tissue homeostasis since removal of cilia could promote as well as suppress Hh-driven BCC depending on the oncogenic context (Wong et al., 2009). This action is not tissue-dependent as it is also observed in other Hh-driven tumors such as MB (Han et al., 2009).

There are three Gli proteins in the mammalian Hh signaling pathway. Among them, Gli2 is the major mediator of Shh signaling during skin development and tumorigenesis (Mill et al., 2003). *Gli2*$^{-/-}$ mice display hair follicle growth arrest similar to *Shh*$^{-/-}$ mutants and overexpression of Gli2 drives BCC development and supports tumor growth (Mill et al., 2003; Hutchin et al., 2005; Grachtchouk et al., 2000). In addition, the level of Gli activity can determine tumor type and latency (Huntziker et al., 2006; Grachtchouk et al., 2001). How Gli2 is regulated in the skin is unclear, however recent studies have demonstrated that

Suppressor of fused (Sufu) and Kif7 are evolutionarily conserved regulators of Gli transcription factors. Sufu, like Ptc, acts as a major negative regulator of the Hh pathway and *in vitro* studies revealed that Sufu inhibits Gli-dependent transcription by anchoring Gli2 in the cytoplasm to prevent its access to the nucleus (Humke et al., 2010; Tukachinsky et al., 2010). Upon Hh stimulus, Gli dissociates from Sufu and translocates freely to the nucleus to activate Hh-target gene transcription (Humke et al., 2010; Tukachinsky et al., 2010). *SUFU* mutations have been identified in patients with sporadic BCC; however, these are accompanied by additional mutations including *PTCH* and *TRP53* (*p53*). Therefore, it is difficult to determine whether *SUFU* mutations are the driver or merely passenger mutations (Reifenberger et al., 2005). Complete ablation of *Sufu* in mice leads to embryonic lethality and there is conflicting data as to whether $Sufu^{+/-}$ mice are prone to skin tumors (Svard et al., 2006; Cooper et al., 2005; Lee et al., 2007). Analysis of *Sufu* deletion specifically in the skin will be useful to resolve this issue. Another regulator of Gli proteins is Kif7, a kinesin molecule that acts predominantly as a negative regulator of the Hh pathway (Cheung et al., 2009; Liem et al., 2009; Endoh-Yamagami et al., 2009). Kif7 is localized to the base of cilia when the pathway is inactive and it translocates to the cilia tip upon pathway activation (Endoh-Yamagami et al., 2009; Liem et al., 2009). Upon Hh stimulus, Kif7 is required for the accumulation of Gli2 and Gli3 to the cilia tip (Endoh-Yamagami et al., 2009; Liem et al., 2009), but the molecular significance of this action has yet to be determined, and whether Kif7 plays a role in the skin remains unknown. Since the activity of the Hh pathway ultimately culminates on the Gli proteins, studying how molecules regulate Gli2 is critical for our understanding of the molecular events of BCC pathogenesis.

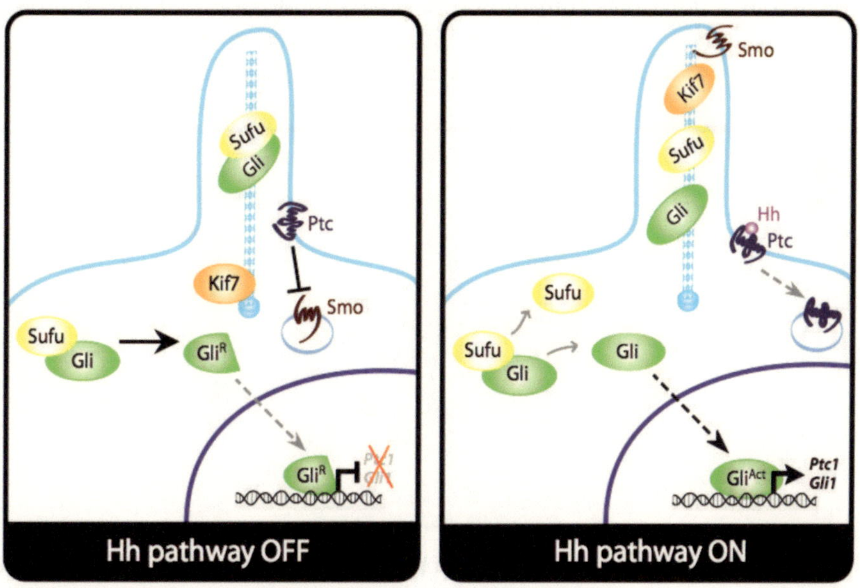

Fig. 1. Vertebrate Hh signal transduction. See text for details.

3. Patched receptors and *Patched* animal models of BCC

Human BCCs are difficult to culture and classical mouse models of skin tumors often develop other skin tumors and not BCC. This has in many ways hampered efforts to understand BCC pathogenesis. It was not until the generation of the *Ptc1*$^{+/-}$ mice that BCC research truly began to advance. *Ptc1*$^{+/-}$ mice display many features of NBCCS and develop BCC (upon ionizing or ultraviolet (UV) radiation) that has many clinical and histochemical features of its human tumor counterparts: slow progression, local invasiveness, and lack of metastasis (Aszterbaum et al., 1999; Mancuso et al., 2004). This model facilitated the identification of both the genetic events and the molecular basis of BCC. Table 1 outlines the current models of BCC using *Ptc* mutant mice. Next, we will describe how the *Ptc1* mutant mouse model revealed the temporal importance of proliferation for BCC formation as well as gave insight into the genetic control, molecular events and the cell of origin of BCC.

3.1 The Patched family members: Patched1 and Patched2

Ptc receptors contain 12 hydrophobic membrane-spanning domains, two large hydrophilic extracellular loops as well as intracellular amino- and carboxyl-terminal regions (Figure 2). The Ptc receptors have a sterol-sensing domain (SSD) and belong to a family of integral-membrane proteins (Kuwabara and Labouesse 2002). SSDs are implicated in vesicle trafficking and cholesterol homeostasis. In addition, the predicted transmembrane topology of Ptc is similar to the resistance nodulation division (RND) family of prototypic bacterial multidrug efflux pumps. RND proteins in bacteria typically transport substrates from the cytoplasm to the extracellular space. How Ptc inhibits Smo is not well understood but it is not likely through direct physical interactions since Ptc can inhibit a large stoichiometric excess of Smo (Taipale et al., 2002). One possibility is that Ptc could function as a molecular transporter for a small molecule that directly binds to or regulates Smo activity. In agreement with this notion, natural and synthetic molecules can modulate the ability of Smo to activate the Hh pathway (Chen et al, 2002).

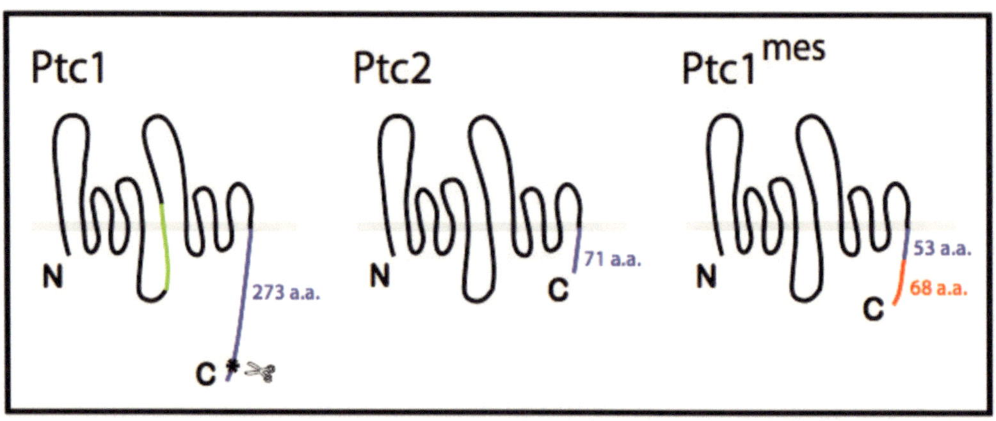

Fig. 2. Topological models of the mouse Ptc receptors. The two large extracellular loops of Ptc receptors bind to the Hh ligands. The CTD of Ptc1 is 273 amino acids in length while the CTD of Ptc2 only extends to 71 amino acids (blue). Green denotes the proposed cyclin B1 interacting domain of Ptc1 (amino acids 690-779) Amino acids 690-779 of Ptc1 is 51% identical to a similar region on Ptc2. Ptc1^{mes} protein retains the first 53 amino acids (blue) of the C-terminal cytoplasmic domain and gains a missence mutation of 68 amino acids (red); therefore, lacks most of its CTD. Predicated caspase-cleavage site (asterisks).

Mutant	Type of mutation	Phenotype	References
Ptc1+/-	Loss of function (in-frame fusion of *lacZ* reporter to exons 1 and 2)	Features of NBCCS and increased susceptibility to spontanous tumor development (RMS and MB) Low frequency of spontanous trichoblastoma-like tumors Enhanced tircholastoma-like tumors and microscopic BCC-like lesions were observed after ultraviolet or ionizing radiation	Goodrich et al., 1997; Aszterbaum et al., 1999;
Ptc1neo67/+	Loss of function (deletion of exons 6 and 7)	Features of NBCCS and increased susceptibiilty to spontanous tumor development (RMS and MB) Non-irradiated mice develop basaloid hyperproliferation in the skin Irradiated mice develop nodular and iniltrative BCC-like tumors	Hahn et al., 1998; Mancuso et al., 2004
Ptc1mes/mes	Deletion of the most C-terminal cytoplasmic domain	Excess skin; basal cell layer hyperplasia and expansion of the epidermal stem cell compartment in adult skin	Makino et al., 2001; Nieuwenhuis et al., 2007
Ptc1flox/flox	Conditional allele	BCC develops when crossed to skin-specific promoters of Cre (K6-Cre, K14-Cre, K5-CrePR1, and Lgr5-CreERT2)	Adolphe et al., 2006 Villani et al., 2010 Kasper et al., 2011
Ptc1D11	Weak allele, effect on gene and protein product is unknown	*Ptc1* homozygous mice are sterile but appears normal	Oro and Higgins, 2003
PtcB6	Polymorphism the C-terminus (T1267N) of *Ptc1* allele found in C57BL/6 background mice compared to FVB/N mice	C57BL/6 mice are resistant to squamouse cell carcinoma induced by activated Ras	Wakabayashi et al., 2007
Ptc2-/-	Truncated *Ptc2* mRNA (deletion of exons 5-17), effect on protein product is unknown	No discernable skin defect; however, *Ptc1* and *Ptc2* compound mutants have increased tumor susceptiblity compared to *Ptc1* mutants	Lee et al., 2006
Ptc2tm1/tm1	Hypomorphic allele (disruption of exon 6), with several truncated *Ptc2* mRNA products produced, effect on protein product is unknown	Male-specific alopecia, ulceration and epidermal hyperplasia with progressing age	Nieuwenhuis et al., 2006

Abbreviations: BCC, basal cell carcinoma; NBCCS, nevoid basal cell carcinoma syndrome; MB, medulloblastoma; RMS, rhabdomyosarcoma

Table 1. Summary of Genetic Analyses of Ptc function in the mouse skin.

There are two *Ptc* genes in vertebrates: *Ptc1* and *Ptc2*. *PTCH2/Ptc2* encodes a protein with 45% identity to *PTCH1/Ptc1* and contains much shorter intracellular amino- and carboxy-terminal regions than Ptc1 (Figure 2). They also differ in the hydrophilic loop between transmembrane domain 6 (TM6) and TM7. Hh ligands bind to the two extracellular loops of PTCH1 and PTCH2 with similar affinity (Carpenter et al., 1998; Marigo et al., 1996). Both Ptc1 and Ptc2 inhibit Hh pathway activity in the absence of ligand, however whether this inhibition is equivalent has not been determined. *PTCH2* mutations were found in some cases of sporadic BCC, and a *PTCH2* germline mutation was identified in a family with NBCCS (Fan et al., 2008; Smyth et al., 1999). This suggests that Ptc2 has a role in development and possibly tumor suppression. We found that *Ptc2*-deficient ($Ptc2^{tm1/tm1}$) mice are viable, fertile and do not develop any obvious developmental defects in Hh-responding tissues, such as the hair follicle, limb, neural tube or testis (Nieuwenhuis et al., 2006). However, with age, adult male $Ptc2^{tm1/tm1}$ mice develop epidermal hyperplasia and hair loss. Ptc2-deficient mice are not cancer prone but, in the $Ptc1^{+/-}$ background, $Ptc2^{+/-}$ and $Ptc2^{-/-}$ mice showed a higher incidence of tumors including BCC when compared to $Ptc1^{+/-}$ mice (Lee et al., 2006). These studies demonstrate that Ptc2 is required during adult skin homeostasis and possesses overlapping functions with Ptc1 in tumor suppression. The divergence of Ptc receptor expression patterns and levels may reflect their unique and overlapping roles during embryogenesis and in maintenance of adult tissues such as the skin (Carpenter et al., 1998; Motoyama et al., 1998; Nieuwenhuis et al., 2006).

3.2 Insights gained from Patched animal models

$Ptc1^{+/-}$ mice in many regards recapitulate the typical pathologies associated with NBCCS, including a higher sensitivity to spontaneous tumorigenesis (Aszterbaum et al., 1999; Goodrich et al., 1996). The vast majorities of these tumors are MB and RMB, and at a low frequency, skin tumors. When these mice are exposed to UV or ionizing radiation, BCC-like lesions form, suggesting that additional genetic alterations, possibly caused by DNA damage, are required to promote BCC progression. Consistent with this notion, human BCC typically occur in sun-exposed areas of the skin and BCC with *PTCH1* mutation are frequently associated with mutations in *p53*, a tumor suppressor gene that is mutated in over 50% of all human tumors (Ponten et al., 1997; Zhang et al., 2001). Furthermore, BCC formation in $Ptc1^{+/-}$ mice was enhanced upon the ablation of *p53* in the skin, suggesting that Ptc1 mutations synergize with the loss of p53 to promote BCC (Wang et al., 2011). Intriguingly, loss of p53 induces the expression of Smo, an obligatory signal transducer of the pathway in the interfollicular epidermis (IFE), where Smo expression is normally not detected (Wang et al., 2011). How p53 contributes to BCC development is unclear but this finding suggests that loss of p53 may promote BCC through its effects on the expression of Hh components. Another genetic signature found in BCC is the loss of heterozygosity (LOH) at the *PTCH1* locus and NBCCS patients with BCC have the remaining somatic wild-type *PTCH1* allele mutated or deleted (Teh et al., 2005). Similarly, LOH at the *Ptc1* locus is observed in tumors of *Ptc1+/-* mice after exposure to UV or ionizing radiation, further illustrating that DNA damaging agents are a strong etiological factor in BCC (Aszterbaum et al., 1999). Whether inactivation of the second allele of *PTCH1* is required for BCC formation could not be conclusively addressed using $Ptc1^{+/-}$ models. Using *Ptc1* conditional knockout mice, it was reported that mice develop BCC only upon biallelic loss of *Ptc1* whereas monoallelic inactivation of *Ptc1* is not sufficient to induce tumorigenesis (Zibat et al., 2009; Kasper et al.,

2011). These studies have revealed that *Ptc1* is a classical tumor suppressor gene and follows Knudson's two hit hypothesis that germline mutation in the *PTCH1* locus requires a "second hit" for tumorigenesis to occur (Knudson 1996).

Interestingly, the frequency of BCC and histological BCC subtypes that develop in $Ptc1^{+/-}$ mice correlates with the phase of the hair follicle cycle at the time of irradiation. In the adult skin, the hair undergoes cyclic nature of active growth (anagen), regression (catagen) and rest (telogen) (Figure 3A). Hair follicle keratinocytes at anagen are highly proliferative since they are required to generate a new follicle at each hair cycle. Shh pathway activation acts as a biological switch for the transition from telogen to anagen. *Shh* is only detectable during anagen and is transcribed asymmetrically in the distal growing tip of the hair follicle, while in the IFE, little to no expression of *Shh* or Hh target genes is detected (Oro and Higgins 2003). During anagen, Hh target genes are expressed in the hair matrix and dermal papilla suggesting that these cells represent Hh-responding cells (Oro and Higgins 2003). As the hair degenerates, *Ptc1* and *Gli1* expression decrease and becomes undetectable at telogen (Oro and Higgins 2003). $Ptc1^{+/-}$ mice irradiated at anagen exhibited more advance tumor growth and much earlier tumor onset than mice irradiated at telogen (Mancuso et al., 2006). This suggests that the hair cycle-induced differences in the proliferation capability of keratinocytes can regulate BCC latency and progression.

Conditional deletion of *Ptc1* in the skin has revealed possible molecular events and pathways involved in BCC. Inactivation of *Ptc1* in the skin induces rapid skin tumor formation without disrupting the expression pattern of Notch signaling components and the nucleo-cytoplasmic distribution of β-catenin, key signaling molecules known to play a role in the skin (Adolphe et al., 2006). Loss of *Ptc1* results in the nuclear accumulation of cell cycle regulators cyclin B1 and cyclin D1, suggesting that Ptc1 functions as a tumor suppressor in the skin in part through regulation of the G1-S and G2-M check points of the cell cycle (Adolphe et al., 2006). Consistent with this finding, Ptc1 has been shown to physically interact with cyclin B1, tethering it in the cytoplasm (Barnes et al., 2001). The authors tested the clinical significance of this interaction by generating a construct that contains a common *PTCH1* mutation found in NBCCS/BCC patients, which lacks the cyclin B1-binding domain (Barnes et al., 2005). Cell culture experiments have shown that $Ptc1^{Q688X}$, a mutant construct encoding a Ptc1 protein truncated at the large intracellular loop, enhances Gli1 activity, promotes proliferation and is non-responsive to Shh treatment (Barnes et al., 2005). Since Gli2 has been shown to promote the transcription of D-type cyclins, nuclear translocation of cyclin D1 is likely a consequence of activated Hh pathway rather than a direct interaction with Ptc1.

Ptc1 has also been shown to inhibit basal cell progenitor expansion possibly through limiting the activity of Insulin-like growth factor binding protein 2 (Igfbp2) (Villani et al, 2010). The function of Igfbp2 in the skin is unknown; however, there is a positive correlation between Igfbp2 expression and human BCC raising the possibility that Igfbp2 is associated with BCC (Villani et al, 2010). Whether the control on Igfbp2 activity is a Ptc1-specific function or a consequence of activated pathway activity remains unknown.

The skin is composed of functionally and biologically distinct units: hair follicle, IFE and the sebaceous gland (Figure 3B). The basal cell layer in the IFE is continuous with the outer root sheath (ORS) of the hair follicle and contains progenitor keratinocytes. Two populations of stem cells are required to maintain skin homeostasis: one that resides in the hair follicle niche, the bulge and the other dispersed in the IFE (Levy et al., 2005). Genetic lineage analysis demonstrated that bulge cells are capable of generating all lineages of the hair follicle to ensure proper tissue homeostasis but only contribute to IFE during wound healing (Levy et al., 2007; Ito et al., 2005). Given that the skin is composed of different cell populations, a key question that arises is what is the cell of origin of BCC? The development of molecular tools was critical to address this question. Using different cell type-specific promoters to drive Cre expression to conditionally express an activating mutation in Smo (SmoM2), Blainpain's group elegantly showed that specifically activating Hh signaling in the long-lived K14+ progenitors of the IFE induces BCC formation (Youssef et al., 2010). In contrast, K15+ cell fate mapping analysis on irradiated $Ptc^{+/-}$ model of BCC revealed that the majority of BCC arose from K15 expressing hair follicle bulge stem cells (Wang et al., 2011). These studies would suggest that both hair follicle stem cells (K15+) and epidermal progenitor cells (K14+) are capable of tumor-initiation and that epidermal cell subpopulations are sensitive to different Hh-driven BCC mutations. Interestingly, cutaneous injury has been shown to influence the cell of origin of BCC. For example, overexpression of SmoM2 in the K15+ bulge cells does not lead to BCC; however, wounding can induce migration of oncogene-expressing bulge cells to the sites of injury to promote BCC formation (Wong and Reiter 2011). Taken together, these studies illustrate that the cell of origin of BCC is context dependent, encompassing both the type of activating mutations and factors involved in wound healing.

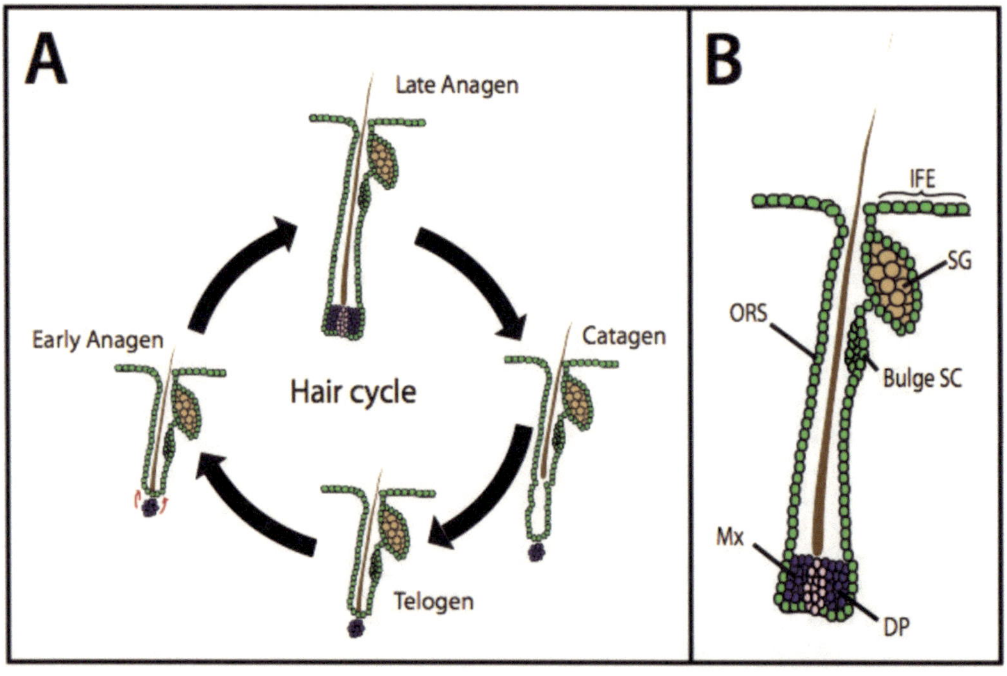

Fig. 3. Adult hair cycle. In the adult skin, the hair follicle constantly degenerates (catagen), rests (telogen) and grows (anagen). Only the non-permanent region of the hair follicle, below the bulge stem cells (SC) participates in these phases of hair cycle. Bulge SCs are located beneath the sebaceous gland (SG). Following telogen, when the dermal papilla (DP) is proximal to the permanent follicle segment, the bulge SC are activated (red arrows) to initiate a new round of hair growth by producing transiently amplifying cells/matrix cells (Mx). The matrix cells will give rise to all differentiated layers of the mature hair follicle.

4. C-terminal domain of Ptc1: Cell survival, cell cycle progression and stem cell maintenance in the epidermis

Besides its ability to inhibit Hh signaling, Ptc1 has been shown to act as a dependence receptor. Dependence receptors promote cell survival when bound to their ligands and induce programmed cell death in the absence of the ligand. Overexpression of Ptc1 results in apoptosis in both cell culture and the neural tube of chick embryos and this can be reversed through addition of Shh ligand (Thibert et al., 2003). The ability of Ptc1 to induce cell death is dependent on a caspase-cleavage site located at Asp 1392, 42 amino acids from the C-terminus of Ptc1 (Figure 2) (Thibert et al., 2003; Mille et al., 2009). Interestingly, Ptc-induced cell death is not affected through expression of Smo, suggesting that Ptc's ability to induce apoptosis is independent of Ptc-Smo transduction. How Ptc transduces this survival signal downstream and whether this is dependent on the Gli transcription factors are unknown.

Interestingly, the majority of *PTCH1* mutations identified in BCC result in premature truncation of the protein (Daya-Grosjean and Couve-Privat 2005). These findings raise the tantalizing possibility that the C-terminal half of *PTCH1* is crucial for tumor suppression. Little is known about the C-terminal domain (CTD) of Ptc1 in the context of skin development and homeostasis. Our group aimed to address these questions by analyzing *Ptc1*^{mes} mice. A spontaneous recessive mutation in *Ptc1, mesenchymal dysplasia* (*mes*) was found in mice containing a missense mutation resulting in a 32bp deletion and a 152 amino acid truncation of the CTD (Figure 2) (Sweet et al., 1996; Makino et al., 2001). It was reported that *Ptc1*$^{mes/mes}$ mice possess excess skin, suggesting that the CTD of Ptc1 is involved in skin development and/or homeostasis (Makino et al., 2001). We found that adult *Ptc1*$^{mes/mes}$ mice have severe epidermal hyperplasia starting as early as postnatal day 12. These mice displayed hyperproliferation of the basal cell population, attributed to increased c-Myc expression, while stratification and apoptosis of the epidermis were not affected. Despite the fact that Ptc1 is a major negative regulator of Hh signaling, *Ptc1*$^{mes/mes}$ mice displayed normal pathway activity in the epidermis, and the Ptc1^{mes} protein maintained similar Shh-binding abilities to wild-type Ptc1. These data suggest that the function of the CTD is independent of Shh pathway/Gli activity. Normally, epidermal stem cells rarely divide and reside in two functionally distinct locations in the skin: the bulge and the IFE. Using BrdU pulse-chase labeling, we found that *Ptc1*$^{mes/mes}$ epidermis exhibited an increase in the number of label-retaining cells (i.e. quiescent stem cells) in the IFE, indicating that the CTD is required for epidermal stem cell maintenance (Figure 4). Despite the persistent hyperplasia phenotype, *Ptc1*$^{mes/mes}$ mice do not develop skin tumors even in response to the DNA damaging effects of radiation (unpublished data). It has been reported that the level of Hh pathway activity determines tumor outcome, ranging from epidermal hyperplasia to BCCs. Therefore we speculate that the lack of tumorigenesis may be attributed to normal Hh pathway activity observed in *Ptc1*$^{mes/mes}$ adult mice. As wounding can contribute to tumor outcome, it would be interesting to determine whether injury can promote tumorigenesis in the *mes* background. Given that *Ptc1*$^{+/-}$ mice are more susceptible to tumorigenesis, whether the *mes* mutation can modulate tumorigenesis of *Ptc1*$^{+/-}$ mice remains to be determined. Together, our study revealed a novel, unexpected role for the CTD of Ptc1 in the regulation of epidermal homeostasis. Furthermore, it highlights a non-canonical function of Ptc1, which appears to be independent of Gli activity.

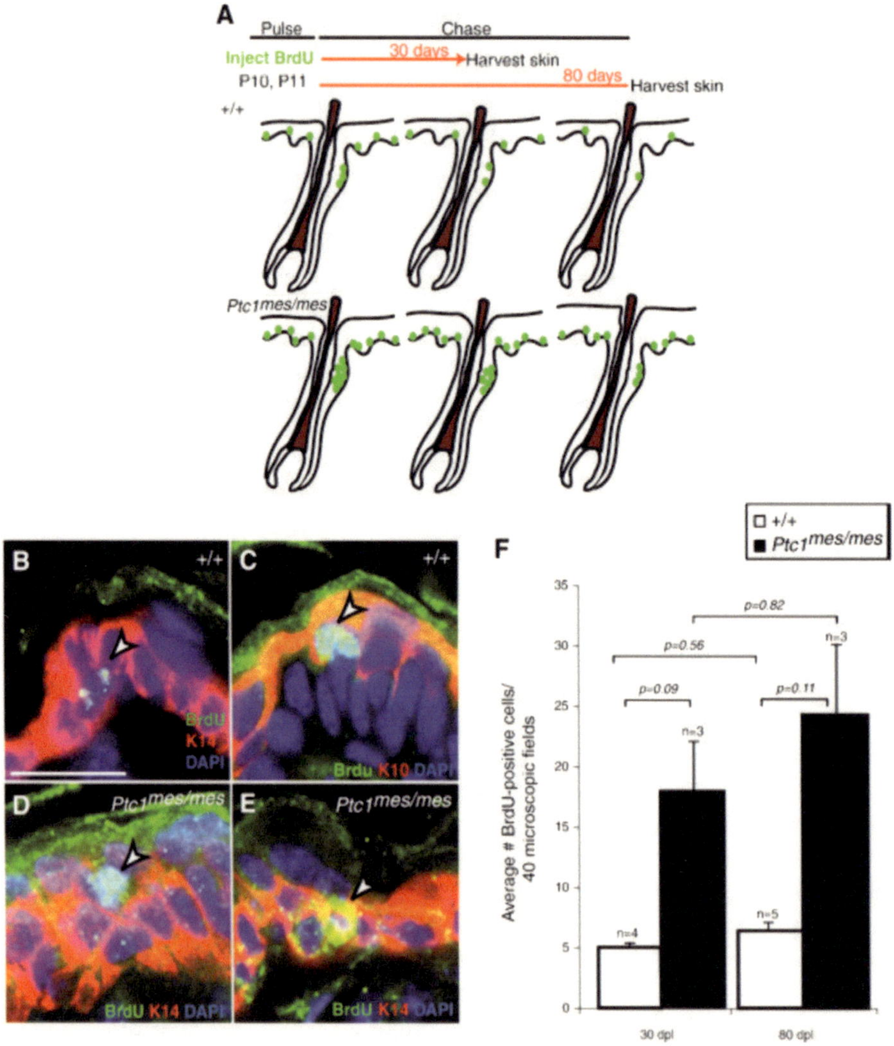

Fig. 4. *Ptc1*$^{mes/mes}$ epidermis exhibits an increase in the number of label-retaining cells. (A) Schematic diagram illustrating pulse-chase experiment. Ten-day-old wild-type and *Ptc1*$^{mes/mes}$ pups received four consecutive BrdU injections at 12-hour intervals to label all mitotic cells. Skin samples were collected 30 and 80 days post-labeling (dpl). (B–E) Basal cells were identified using K-14/BrdU double labelling and are considered to be label-retaining interfollicular epidermal stem cells (B, D, E; arrowheads). Suprabasal cells were identified using K-10/BrdU double labeling. These cells were not considered to be interfollicular stem cells and were not counted (C; arrowhead). (D, E) BrdU/K-14-double positive cells could be detected at 30 (D) and 80 (E) dpl in wild-type and *Ptc1*$^{mes/mes}$ skin. (F) At 30 days, skin showed a 3.6-fold increase in BrdU/K14-double positive cells. A 3.3-fold increase was observed at 80 dpl. Data represent the mean ± SEM. Scale bars = 50 μm. Reprinted from Developmental Biology, E.N., P.C.B., S.M., C.-c. H., Epidermal hyperplasia and expansion of the interfollicular stem cell compartment in mutant mice with C-terminal truncation of *Patched1*, 308, 547-560, © 2007, with permission from Elsevier.

5. Conclusion and future prospective

The establishment of *Ptc* mutant mouse models of BCC has given us critical insight into the genetic underpinnings and the molecular events that drive BCC formation. We described here that the tumor suppressor Ptc1 is a multifaceted protein that is not solely dedicated to repressing the Hh pathway. By attempting to understand BCC biology using the *Ptc1* mouse model, researchers have serendipitously stumbled upon the non-canonical functions of Ptc1. In the neural tube, Shh can act as a chemical cue to guide commissural axons independent of Gli transcription factors, further illustrating that Gli activity is not always coupled to the Shh-Ptc module (Okada et al., 2006; Yam et al., 2009). Interestingly, the non-canonical actions of Ptc1 can be traced to its C-terminal domain, which is largely absent in Ptc2, suggesting a functional divergence between the Ptc family of receptors.

Our group found that the CTD of Ptc1 is important in stem cell homeostasis of the IFE, identifying Ptc1 as a pivotal switch between quiescence or cell cycle progression (Nieuwenhuis et al., 2007). The molecular events mediating this outcome remain unclear. We speculate that the CTD of Ptc1 might act as a docking site for regulatory proteins required for stem cell maintenance. Determining these potential binding partners could help decipher the atypical functions of Ptc1. Mutations of the *PTCH1* locus in BCC typically display a truncating mutation in one allele and a deletion on the other (Reichrath 2006). Further analyses on the monoallelic loss of *Ptc1* in conjunction with *Ptc1* point mutations will be necessary to recapitulate the molecular events leading to BCC pathogenesis, which cannot be uncovered using current *Ptc* mouse models.

6. References

Adolphe, C., R. Hetherington, T. Ellis & B. Wainwright (2006) Patched1 functions as a gatekeeper by promoting cell cycle progression. *Cancer Res,* 66, 2081-8.

Aszterbaum, M., J. Epstein, A. Oro, V. Douglas, P. E. LeBoit, M. P. Scott & E. H. Epstein, Jr. (1999) Ultraviolet and ionizing radiation enhance the growth of BCCs and trichoblastomas in patched heterozygous knockout mice. *Nat Med,* 5, 1285-91.

Barnes, E. A., K. J. Heidtman & D. J. Donoghue (2005) Constitutive activation of the shh-ptc1 pathway by a patched1 mutation identified in BCC. *Oncogene,* 24, 902-15.

Barnes, E. A., M. Kong, V. Ollendorff & D. J. Donoghue (2001) Patched1 interacts with cyclin B1 to regulate cell cycle progression. *EMBO J,* 20, 2214-23.

Carpenter, D., D. M. Stone, J. Brush, A. Ryan, M. Armanini, G. Frantz, A. Rosenthal & F. J. de Sauvage (1998) Characterization of two patched receptors for the vertebrate hedgehog protein family. *Proc Natl Acad Sci U S A,* 95, 13630-4.

Chen, J. K., J. Taipale, K. E. Young, T. Maiti & P. A. Beachy (2002) Small molecule modulation of Smoothened activity. *Proc Natl Acad Sci U S A,* 99, 14071-6.

Cheung, H. O., X. Zhang, A. Ribeiro, R. Mo, S. Makino, V. Puviindran, K. K. Law, J. Briscoe & C. C. Hui (2009) The kinesin protein Kif7 is a critical regulator of Gli transcription factors in mammalian hedgehog signaling. *Sci Signal,* 2, ra29.

Cooper, A. F., K. P. Yu, M. Brueckner, L. L. Brailey, L. Johnson, J. M. McGrath & A. E. Bale (2005) Cardiac and CNS defects in a mouse with targeted disruption of suppressor of fused. *Development,* 132, 4407-17.

Daya-Grosjean, L. & S. Couve-Privat (2005) Sonic hedgehog signaling in basal cell carcinomas. *Cancer Lett,* 225, 181-92.

Endoh-Yamagami, S., M. Evangelista, D. Wilson, X. Wen, J. W. Theunissen, K. Phamluong, M. Davis, S. J. Scales, M. J. Solloway, F. J. de Sauvage & A. S. Peterson (2009) The mammalian Cos2 homolog Kif7 plays an essential role in modulating Hh signal transduction during development. *Curr Biol,* 19, 1320-6.

Fan, Z., J. Li, J. Du, H. Zhang, Y. Shen, C. Y. Wang & S. Wang (2008) A missense mutation in PTCH2 underlies dominantly inherited NBCCS in a Chinese family. *J Med Genet,* 45, 303-8.

Goetz, S. C. & K. V. Anderson (2010) The primary cilium: a signalling centre during vertebrate development. *Nat Rev Genet,* 11, 331-44.

Goodrich, L. V., R. L. Johnson, L. Milenkovic, J. A. McMahon & M. P. Scott (1996) Conservation of the hedgehog/patched signaling pathway from flies to mice: induction of a mouse patched gene by Hedgehog. *Genes Dev,* 10, 301-12.

Gorlin, R. J. & R. W. Goltz (1960) Multiple nevoid basal-cell epithelioma, jaw cysts and bifid rib. A syndrome. *N Engl J Med,* 262, 908-12.

Gorlin, R. J. (2004) Nevoid basal cell carcinoma (Gorlin) syndrome. *Genet Med,* 6, 530-9.

Grachtchouk, M., J. Pero, S. H. Yang, A. N. Ermilov, L. E. Michael, A. Wang, D. Wilbert, R. M. Patel, J. Ferris, J. Diener, M. Allen, S. Lim, L. J. Syu, M. Verhaegen & A. A. Dlugosz (2011) Basal cell carcinomas in mice arise from hair follicle stem cells and multiple epithelial progenitor populations. *J Clin Invest,* 121, 1768-81.

Grachtchouk, M., R. Mo, S. Yu, X. Zhang, H. Sasaki, C. C. Hui & A. A. Dlugosz (2000) Basal cell carcinomas in mice overexpressing Gli2 in skin. *Nat Genet,* 24, 216-7.

Grachtchouk, V., M. Grachtchouk, L. Lowe, T. Johnson, L. Wei, A. Wang, F. de Sauvage & A. A. Dlugosz (2003) The magnitude of hedgehog signaling activity defines skin tumor phenotype. *EMBO J,* 22, 2741-51.

Hahn, H., C. Wicking, P. G. Zaphiropoulous, M. R. Gailani, S. Shanley, A. Chidambaram, I. Vorechovsky, E. Holmberg, A. B. Unden, S. Gillies, K. Negus, I. Smyth, C. Pressman, D. J. Leffell, B. Gerrard, A. M. Goldstein, M. Dean, R. Toftgard, G. Chenevix-Trench, B. Wainwright & A. E. Bale (1996) Mutations of the human homolog of Drosophila patched in the nevoid basal cell carcinoma syndrome. *Cell,* 85, 841-51.

Hahn, H., L. Wojnowski, A.M. Zimmer, J. Hall, G. Miller & A. Zimmer (1998) Rhabdomyosarcomas and radiation hypersensitivity in a mouse model of Gorlin syndrome. *Nat Med,* 4, 619-22.

Han, Y. G., H. J. Kim, A. A. Dlugosz, D. W. Ellison, R. J. Gilbertson & A. Alvarez-Buylla (2009) Dual and opposing roles of primary cilia in medulloblastoma development. *Nat Med,* 15, 1062-5.

Huangfu, D. & K. V. Anderson (2005) Cilia and Hedgehog responsiveness in the mouse. *Proc Natl Acad Sci U S A,* 102, 11325-30.

Humke, E. W., K. V. Dorn, L. Milenkovic, M. P. Scott & R. Rohatgi (2010) The output of Hedgehog signaling is controlled by the dynamic association between Suppressor of Fused and the Gli proteins. *Genes Dev,* 24, 670-82.

Huntzicker, E. G., I. S. Estay, H. Zhen, L. A. Lokteva, P. K. Jackson & A. E. Oro (2006) Dual degradation signals control Gli protein stability and tumor formation. *Genes Dev,* 20, 276-81.

Hutchin, M. E., M. S. Kariapper, M. Grachtchouk, A. Wang, L. Wei, D. Cummings, J. Liu, L. E. Michael, A. Glick & A. A. Dlugosz (2005) Sustained Hedgehog signaling is required for basal cell carcinoma proliferation and survival: conditional skin tumorigenesis recapitulates the hair growth cycle. *Genes Dev,* 19, 214-23.

Ito, M., Y. Liu, Z. Yang, J. Nguyen, F. Liang, R. J. Morris & G. Cotsarelis (2005) Stem cells in the hair follicle bulge contribute to wound repair but not to homeostasis of the epidermis. *Nat Med,* 11, 1351-4.

Jiang, J. & C. C. Hui (2008) Hedgehog signaling in development and cancer. *Dev Cell,* 15, 801-12.

Johnson, R. L., A. L. Rothman, J. Xie, L. V. Goodrich, J. W. Bare, J. M. Bonifas, A. G. Quinn, R. M. Myers, D. R. Cox, E. H. Epstein, Jr. & M. P. Scott (1996) Human homolog of patched, a candidate gene for the basal cell nevus syndrome. *Science,* 272, 1668-71.

Kasper, M., V. Jaks, A. Are, A. Bergstrom, A. Schwager, N. Barker & R. Toftgard (2011) Wounding enhances epidermal tumorigenesis by recruiting hair follicle keratinocytes. *Proc Natl Acad Sci U S A,* 108, 4099-104.

Knudson, A. G. (1996) Hereditary cancer: two hits revisited. *J Cancer Res Clin Oncol,* 122, 135-40.

Kuwabara, P. E. & M. Labouesse (2002) The sterol-sensing domain: multiple families, a unique role? *Trends Genet,* 18, 193-201.

Lee, Y., H. L. Miller, H. R. Russell, K. Boyd, T. Curran & P. J. McKinnon (2006) Patched2 modulates tumorigenesis in patched1 heterozygous mice. *Cancer Res,* 66, 6964-71.

Lee, Y., R. Kawagoe, K. Sasai, Y. Li, H. R. Russell, T. Curran & P. J. McKinnon (2007) Loss of suppressor-of-fused function promotes tumorigenesis. *Oncogene,* 26, 6442-7.

Levy, V., C. Lindon, B. D. Harfe & B. A. Morgan (2005) Distinct stem cell populations regenerate the follicle and interfollicular epidermis. *Dev Cell,* 9, 855-61.

Levy, V., C. Lindon, Y. Zheng, B. D. Harfe & B. A. Morgan (2007) Epidermal stem cells arise from the hair follicle after wounding. *FASEB J,* 21, 1358-66.

Liem, K. F., Jr., M. He, P. J. Ocbina & K. V. Anderson (2009) Mouse Kif7/Costal2 is a cilia-associated protein that regulates Sonic hedgehog signaling. *Proc Natl Acad Sci U S A,* 106, 13377-82.

Liu, A., B. Wang & L. A. Niswander (2005) Mouse intraflagellar transport proteins regulate both the activator and repressor functions of Gli transcription factors. *Development,* 132, 3103-11.

Makino, S., H. Masuya, J. Ishijima, Y. Yada & T. Shiroishi (2001) A spontaneous mouse mutation, mesenchymal dysplasia (mes), is caused by a deletion of the most C-terminal cytoplasmic domain of patched (ptc). *Dev Biol,* 239, 95-106.

Mancuso, M., S. Leonardi, M. Tanori, E. Pasquali, M. Pierdomenico, S. Rebessi, V. Di Majo, V. Covelli, S. Pazzaglia & A. Saran (2006) Hair cycle-dependent basal cell carcinoma tumorigenesis in Ptc1neo67/+ mice exposed to radiation. *Cancer Res,* 66, 6606-14.

Mancuso, M., S. Pazzaglia, M. Tanori, H. Hahn, P. Merola, S. Rebessi, M. J. Atkinson, V. Di Majo, V. Covelli & A. Saran (2004) Basal cell carcinoma and its development: insights from radiation-induced tumors in Ptch1-deficient mice. *Cancer Res,* 64, 934-41.

Marigo, V., R. A. Davey, Y. Zuo, J. M. Cunningham & C. J. Tabin (1996) Biochemical evidence that patched is the Hedgehog receptor. *Nature,* 384, 176-9.

May, S. R., A. M. Ashique, M. Karlen, B. Wang, Y. Shen, K. Zarbalis, J. Reiter, J. Ericson & A. S. Peterson (2005) Loss of the retrograde motor for IFT disrupts localization of Smo to cilia and prevents the expression of both activator and repressor functions of Gli. *Dev Biol,* 287, 378-89.

Mill, P., R. Mo, H. Fu, M. Grachtchouk, P. C. Kim, A. A. Dlugosz & C. C. Hui (2003) Sonic hedgehog-dependent activation of Gli2 is essential for embryonic hair follicle development. *Genes Dev,* 17, 282-94.

Mille, F., C. Thibert, J. Fombonne, N. Rama, C. Guix, H. Hayashi, V. Corset, J. C. Reed & P. Mehlen (2009) The Patched dependence receptor triggers apoptosis through a DRAL-caspase-9 complex. *Nat Cell Biol,* 11, 739-46.

Motoyama, J., H. Heng, M. A. Crackower, T. Takabatake, K. Takeshima, L. C. Tsui & C. Hui (1998) Overlapping and non-overlapping Ptch2 expression with Shh during mouse embryogenesis. *Mech Dev,* 78, 81-4.

Nieuwenhuis, E., J. Motoyama, P. C. Barnfield, Y. Yoshikawa, X. Zhang, R. Mo, M. A. Crackower & C. C. Hui (2006) Mice with a targeted mutation of patched2 are viable but develop alopecia and epidermal hyperplasia. *Mol Cell Biol,* 26, 6609-22.

Nieuwenhuis, E., P. C. Barnfield, S. Makino & C.-c. Hui (2007) Epidermal hyperplasia and expansion of the interfollicular stem cell compartment in mutant mice with a C-terminal truncation of Patched1. *Dev Biol,* 308, 547-60.

Okada, A., F. Charron, S. Morin, D. S. Shin, K. Wong, P. J. Fabre, M. Tessier-Lavigne & S. K. McConnell (2006) Boc is a receptor for sonic hedgehog in the guidance of commissural axons. *Nature,* 444, 369-73.

Oro, A. E. & K. Higgins (2003) Hair cycle regulation of Hedgehog signal reception. *Dev Biol,* 255, 238-48.

Oro, A. E., K. M. Higgins, Z. Hu, J. M. Bonifas, E. H. Epstein, Jr. & M. P. Scott (1997) Basal cell carcinomas in mice overexpressing sonic hedgehog. *Science,* 276, 817-21.

Ponten, F., C. Berg, A. Ahmadian, Z. P. Ren, M. Nister, J. Lundeberg, M. Uhlen & J. Ponten (1997) Molecular pathology in basal cell cancer with p53 as a genetic marker. *Oncogene,* 15, 1059-67.

Reichrath, J. 2006. *Molecular mechanisms of basal cell and squamous cell carcinomas.* Georgetown, Tex. New York, N.Y.: Landes Bioscience/Eurekah.com; Springer Science+Business Media.

Reifenberger, J., M. Wolter, C. B. Knobbe, B. Kohler, A. Schonicke, C. Scharwachter, K. Kumar, B. Blaschke, T. Ruzicka & G. Reifenberger (2005) Somatic mutations in the PTCH, SMOH, SUFUH and TP53 genes in sporadic basal cell carcinomas. *Br J Dermatol,* 152, 43-51.

Ruiz i Altaba, A. 2006. *Hedgehog-gli signaling in human disease.* Georgetown, Tex. New York, N.Y.: Landes Bioscience/Eurekah.com; Springer Science+Business Media.

Smyth, I., M. A. Narang, T. Evans, C. Heimann, Y. Nakamura, G. Chenevix-Trench, T. Pietsch, C. Wicking & B. J. Wainwright (1999) Isolation and characterization of human patched 2 (PTCH2), a putative tumour suppressor gene inbasal cell carcinoma and medulloblastoma on chromosome 1p32. *Hum Mol Genet,* 8, 291-7.

Svard, J., K. Heby-Henricson, M. Persson-Lek, B. Rozell, M. Lauth, A. Bergstrom, J. Ericson, R. Toftgard & S. Teglund (2006) Genetic elimination of Suppressor of fused reveals an essential repressor function in the mammalian Hedgehog signaling pathway. *Dev Cell,* 10, 187-97.

Sweet, H. O., R.T. Bronson, L. R. Donahue & M. T. Davisson (1996) Mesenchymal dysplasia: A recessive mutation on chromosome 13 of the mouse. *J Hered,* 87, 87–95.

Taipale, J., M. K. Cooper, T. Maiti & P. A. Beachy (2002) Patched acts catalytically to suppress the activity of Smoothened. *Nature,* 418, 892-7.

Teh, M. T., D. Blaydon, T. Chaplin, N. J. Foot, S. Skoulakis, M. Raghavan, C. A. Harwood, C. M. Proby, M. P. Philpott, B. D. Young & D. P. Kelsell (2005) Genomewide single nucleotide polymorphism microarray mapping in basal cell carcinomas unveils uniparental disomy as a key somatic event. *Cancer Res,* 65, 8597-603.

Thibert, C., M. A. Teillet, F. Lapointe, L. Mazelin, N. M. Le Douarin & P. Mehlen (2003) Inhibition of neuroepithelial patched-induced apoptosis by sonic hedgehog. *Science,* 301, 843-6.

Tukachinsky, H., L. V. Lopez & A. Salic (2010) A mechanism for vertebrate Hedgehog signaling: recruitment to cilia and dissociation of SuFu-Gli protein complexes. *J Cell Biol,* 191, 415-28.

Villani, R. M., C. Adolphe, J. Palmer, M. J. Waters & B. J. Wainwright (2010) Patched1 inhibits epidermal progenitor cell expansion and basal cell carcinoma formation by limiting Igfbp2 activity. *Cancer Prev Res (Phila),* 3, 1222-34.

Wakabayshi, Y., J. H. Mao, K. Brown, M. Girardi & A. Balmain (2007) Promotion of Hras-induced squamous carcinomas by a polymorphic variant of the Patched gene in FVB mice. Nature, 445, 761-765.

Wang, G. Y., J. Wang, M. L. Mancianti & E. H. Epstein, Jr. (2011) Basal cell carcinomas arise from hair follicle stem cells in Ptch1(+/-) mice. *Cancer Cell,* 19, 114-24.

Wong, S. Y. & J. F. Reiter (2011) Wounding mobilizes hair follicle stem cells to form tumors. *Proc Natl Acad Sci U S A,* 108, 4093-8.

Wong, S. Y., A. D. Seol, P. L. So, A. N. Ermilov, C. K. Bichakjian, E. H. Epstein, Jr., A. A. Dlugosz & J. F. Reiter (2009) Primary cilia can both mediate and suppress Hedgehog pathway-dependent tumorigenesis. *Nat Med,* 15, 1055-61.

Xie, J., M. Murone, S. M. Luoh, A. Ryan, Q. Gu, C. Zhang, J. M. Bonifas, C. W. Lam, M. Hynes, A. Goddard, A. Rosenthal, E. H. Epstein, Jr. & F. J. de Sauvage (1998) Activating Smoothened mutations in sporadic basal-cell carcinoma. *Nature,* 391, 90-2.

Yam, P. T., S. D. Langlois, S. Morin & F. Charron (2009) Sonic hedgehog guides axons through a noncanonical, Src-family-kinase-dependent signaling pathway. *Neuron,* 62, 349-62.

Youssef, K. K., A. Van Keymeulen, G. Lapouge, B. Beck, C. Michaux, Y. Achouri, P. A. Sotiropoulou & C. Blanpain (2010) Identification of the cell lineage at the origin of basal cell carcinoma. *Nat Cell Biol,* 12, 299-305.

Zhang, H., X. L. Ping, P. K. Lee, X. L. Wu, Y. J. Yao, M. J. Zhang, D. N. Silvers, D. Ratner, R. Malhotra, M. Peacocke & H. C. Tsou (2001) Role of PTCH and p53 genes in early-onset basal cell carcinoma. *Am J Pathol,* 158, 381-5.

Zibat, A., A. Uhmann, F. Nitzki, M. Wijgerde, A. Frommhold, T. Heller, V. Armstrong, L. Wojnowski, L. Quintanilla-Martinez, J. Reifenberger, W. Schulz-Schaeffer & H. Hahn (2009) Time-point and dosage of gene inactivation determine the tumor spectrum in conditional Ptch knockouts. *Carcinogenesis,* 30, 918-26.

4

The Role of Cytokines and Chemokines in the Development of Basal Cell Carcinoma

Eijun Itakura
Department of Pathology and Laboratory Medicine,
David Geffen School of Medicine at UCLA, Los Angeles, California
USA

1. Introduction

The immune system plays an important role in surveillance against tumor development, and it is widely known that cancer cells protect themselves against the host's anti-tumor immune defense. Cancer cells have several means of evading the antitumor immunity, one of which is the production of immune modulators such as cytokines and chemokines. These factors can either promote or block immune responses. Many of these molecules are used by cancer cells to promote tumor progression including cell proliferation, cell migration, matrix remodeling, immune suppression and angiogenesis. On the other hand, some molecules are involved in immunotherapeutics for the purpose of enhancing and modifying antitumor immune responses.

In basal cell carcinoma (BCC), several cytokines and chemokines and their receptors are associated with the development of this cutaneous cancer. There are varying degrees of inflammation in BCC. The majority of peritumor inflammatory cells are lymphocytes and most are T cells (1). It has been proposed that the tumor microenvironment of BCC is generally Th2 dominant. T regulatory cells and immature dendritic cells mediated by Th2 cytokines cause immunosuppression and decreased immunity to BCC (2). Tumor-associated macrophages (TAM), which are polarized to M2 type, are associated with tumor invasion and angiogenesis in BCC (3). In this chapter, we focus on cytokines and chemokines which may influence and enhance these immunosuppressive networks.

2. IL-6

Interleukin-6 (IL-6) is a pro-inflammatory cytokine, which can induce tumor progression by manipulating immune responses in the tumor microenvironment. IL-6 is directly related to epidermal hyperproliferation in psoriasis (4). There are many experimental evidences that IL-6 is associated with BCC. Overexpression of IL-6 in BCC cell lines increases anti-apoptotic activity and tumorigenic potency (5). The phosphotidyl inositol 3-kinase (PI3K)/Akt signal pathway is involved in such anti-apoptosis (6). On the other hand, IL-6 induces bFGF-dependent angiogenesis in BCC cell line via JAK/STAT3 and PI3k/Akt pathways (7). IL-6 is also involved in CXCL-12 (SDF-1)-enhanced angiogenesis via activating ERK1/2 and NF-κB (8). IL-6 expression is associated with a significant increase of IL-8 (CXCL8) expression in

BCC (9, 10), one of which functions is tumor angiogenesis. The expression of these two cytokines shows a significant positive correlation (10).

A single nucleotide polymorphism (SNP) in the promoter regions of IL-6 gene (*IL6*) is associated with the risk of BCC. The promoter region of *IL6* contains several SNPs, including -634G>C, -597G>A and -174G>C. It has been reported that *IL6* -597 G>A is significantly associated with BCC risk (11). However, others reported that there was no difference for genotype distributions of SNPs in the promoter region of *IL6* between the BCC cases and controls, while linkage disequilibrium was observed between the -174 and -597 alleles in the *IL6* (12).

3. IL-10

Interleukin-10 (IL-10) is a major immunosuppressive cytokine that plays a critical regulatory role in several areas of the immune system. It contributes to immunosuppression in the tumor microenvironment and may render it permissive for infiltration of cancer cells. IL-10 is upregulated in both melanoma (13-15) and non-melanoma skin cancer including BCC (2, 16, 17). The presence of IL-10 in BCC is associated with the lack of expression of HLA-DR, ICAM-1, CD40 and CD80 and the inconsistent expression of HLA-ABC in BCC (17). BCC is regarded as an indolent (slow growing) cancer with limited metastatic potential. While IL-10 expression by melanoma cells correlates with melanoma progression and development of metastatic competence (18), there is no clear correlation between IL-10 expression and tumor invasiveness of BCC. IL-10 can be detected by both aggressive BCC and nonaggressive BCC such as superficial BCC. However, there are discrepant results regarding IL-10 expression in superficial BCC. Urosevic *et al.* found that superficial BCC cells were uniformly negative for IL-10 expression at baseline and showed little change after imiquimod treatment (19).

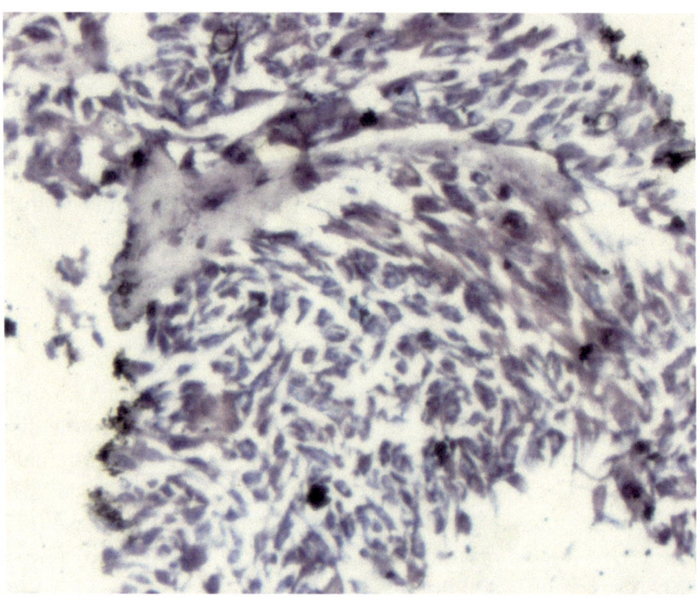

Fig. 1. IL-10 mRNA is expressed by tumor cells in basal cell carcinoma (blue/purple color, RT *in situ* PCR).

SNP in the promoter regions of IL-10 gene (*IL10*) is associated with the risk of BCC. *IL10* -1082G>A is detected in BCC (12), and this polymorphism, as well as tumor necrosis factor-alpha (TNF-α) gene *TNF* -308G>A polymorphism, is more prevalent in aggressive BCC (20). However, others reported that there was no significant association between BCC and *IL10* -1082 (11).

4. CXCL12 and CXCR4

CXCL12 (SDF-1) is a proinflammatory chemokine produced in response to inflammatory stimuli. This chemokine functions as a chemoattractant for lymphocytes. CXCL12 also plays an important role in tumor angiogenesis through binding to its receptor, CXCR4. CXCR4 expression enhances tumorigenesis and angiogenesis in BCC. Such CXCL12-enhanced angiogenesis involves the ERK1/2 and NF-κB pathways mediated by IL-6 (8). CXCR4 is especially expressed in noduloulcerative and sclerosing types of BCC and is associated with more aggressive behavior (21). CXCL12 directs BCC invasion by upregulating gelatinase activity of matrix metalloproteinase-13 (MMP-13). The transcriptional regulation of MMP-13 by CXCL12 is mediated by phosphorylation of ERK1/2 and c-Jun/AP-1 activation (22). CXCL12 also upregulates several angiogenesis-associated genes including interferon alpha-inducible protein 27 (IFI27), bone morphogenetic protein 6 (BMP6) and cyclooxygenase 2 (COX-2) (8).

5. CXCL9, CXCL10, CXCL11 and CXCR3

CXCL9 (MIG), CXCL10 (IP-10) and CXCL11 (I-TAC) are chemokines that are induced by interferon during inflammatory responses. These chemokines bind to a common receptor, CXCR3. They can promote chemotaxis of activated T cells and NK cells through binding to CXCR3. The most recent attention has been given to the role of these chemokines in tumorigenesis of BCC. It has been reported that CXCL9, CXCL10, CXCL11, and their receptor CXCR3 are significantly upregulated in BCC. CXCR3, CXCL10, and CXCL11, but not CXCL9, colocalize with keratin 17, which is a BCC keratinocyte marker. Exposure of BCC cells to CXCL11 *in vitro* enhances keratinocyte cell proliferation (23). CXCL9, CXCL10 and CXCL11 promote expression of functional indoleamine 2,3-dioxygenase (IDO), which also colocalizes with keratin 17 (24). Thus, CXCR3 and its ligands may be important in tumorigenesis of BCC.

6. IL-8 (CXCL8)

Interleukin-8 (IL-8, CXCL8) is a chemokine produced by inflammatory cells and other cell types. This chemokine is one of the major mediators of the inflammatory response. It functions as a chemoattractant, but is also known as an angiogenic factor. IL-8 is associated with tumor angiogenesis in many solid tumors. It has been reported IL-8 is highly expressed in BCC (25). As described earlier in this chapter, IL-8 expression is associated with a significant increase of IL-6 expression in BCC (9, 10), and is positively correlated with IL-6 expression (10). However, the detailed mechanisms of IL-8 involved in the development of BCC are not fully understood.

7. CCL27

CCL27 is a chemokine that functions as a chemoattractant by interacting with its receptor, CCR10. This chemokine regulates T cell homing under homeostatic and inflammatory conditions, and plays a role in T cell-mediated inflammation of the skin. In BCC, the downregulating of CCL27 expression is associated with tumor immune escape. A significant decrease in CCL27 expression is also observed in squamous cell carcinoma and actinic keratosis. These skin tumors may evade T cell-mediated antitumor immune responses by down-regulating the expression of CCL27 through the activation of epidermal growth factor receptor (EGFR)-Ras-MAPK-signaling pathways (26).

8. IFN-γ

Interferon-gamma (IFN-γ) is a cytokine that is critical for immune responses against cancer. IFN-γ binding to the receptor activates the JAK-STAT pathway. In BCC, The expression of IFN-γ receptor is significantly decreased on the cancer cells compared with the overlying epidermis. The absence or paucity of IFN-γ receptor and the absence of intercellular adhesion molecule-1 (ICAM-1) may explain the lack of tumor-infiltrating cells and the lack of an active cell-mediated immune response in BCC (27).

On the other hand, Th1 cytokines including IFN-γ play a role in spontaneously regressing BCC. Some cases of BCC may show spontaneous regression in the absence of therapy. Such spontaneous regression is mediated by activated CD4+ T cells, and IFN-γ is elevated in actively regressing BCC (28). There is a significantly increased number of CD4+ T cells infiltrating regressing tumors, and the expression of IL-2 receptor, which is an early activation marker for T cells is also increased (29). Abundant CD8+ T cells and interferon signal transduction is associated with partial host antitumor response (2).

Imiquimod has been shown to be efficacious as a topical treatment for BCC. Imiquimod is a Toll-like receptor 7 (TLR7) agonist, which induces interferon and other cytokines through the immune system and stimulates innate and adaptive cell-mediated immunity. Clinical studies have demonstrated clinical and histological clearance of superficial BCC after treatment with imiquimod 5% cream (30-32). Imiquimod treatment is associated with the early appearance of lymphocytes and macrophages. This early response tends to be a mixed cellular response of CD4 cells, activated dendritic cells and macrophages, with later infiltration by CD8 T cells (33). Application of imiquimod induces a cascade of Th1 cytokines including IFN-α, TNF-α, IL-1α, IL-12, and IFN-γ, with profound effects on innate and adaptive immunity and on immunologic memory and antigen presentation. IFN-γ is produced by CD4 and CD8 T cells. IFN-γ is associated with the enhanced expression of ICAM-1, promoting the influx of immune cells. Imiquimod treatment also induces a massive increase in macrophage peritumoral and intratumoral infiltration (19). Thus, the TLR7-agonist plays an important role in inducing a lymphocytic infiltrate by promoting specific Th1 cellular immune response capable of eliminating cancer cells (34).

9. FasL (CD95L) and Fas (CD95)

Fas ligand (FasL, CD95L) belongs to the tumor necrosis factor (TNF) family. FasL binds to its receptor, Fas (CD95), and induces apoptosis. Apoptosis via FasL/Fas pathway plays an important role in the regulation of the immune system. FasL expressed by cacncer cells induces apoptosis of infiltrating lymphocytes and they can evade immune surveillance, contributing to cancer progression. BCC has been reported to lack Fas expression (19, 35), while they commonly retain the expression of FasL (36). In normal skin, Fas is expressed by keratinocytes in the basal layer. Fas expression is up-regulated in chronically sun-damaged skin. Actinic keratosis does not express Fas. Squamous cell carcinoma focally expresses Fas at the sites of contact with lymphocytes (35).

It has been suggested that BCC can evade host immune surveillance by expressing FasL (37). However, different results were obtained for the FasL expression in BCC (19, 38, 39), and the issue of FasL expression in BCC is still debatable. After imiquimod treatment, the infiltrating cells demonstrate an increase in Fas/FasL expression, while Fas expression by BCC cells remains unaffected and FasL expression demonstrates either an increase or a decrease in different cases (19). After intralesional IFN-α treatment, BCC cells become Fas-positive with signs of tumor regression as a result of tumor cell apoptosis (36). Thus, Fas/FasL pathway may be associated with tumor regression by such treatments.

Substance	**Alternative name**	**Receptor**	**Action**
IL-6		IL6R (CD126)	Anti-apoptotic activity
IL-8	CXCL8	IL8RA (CXCR1, CD181); IL8RB (CXCR2, CD182)	Tumor angiogenesis
IL-10		IL10RA (CDw210a); IL10RB (CDw210b)	Immune suppression
CXCL9	MIG	CXCR3 (CD183)	Tumorigenesis
CXCL10	IP-10	CXCR3 (CD183)	Tumorigenesis
CXCL11	I-TAC	CXCR3 (CD183)	Tumorigenesis
CXCL12	SDF-1	CXCR4 (CD184)	Tumor angiogenesis; stromal invasion
CCL27	CTACK, ILC, ESKine	CCR10	Immune escape by down-regulation of CCL27
IFN-γ		IFNGR1 (CD119); IFNGR2	Tumor regression; immune escape by down-regulation of IFN-γ receptor
FasL	CD95L	Fas (CD95)	Immune escape

Table 1. Cytokines and chemokines in the pathogenesis of Basal Cell Carcinoma.

10. Conclusions

There is much more work to be done in order to adequately characterize the clinical significance of cytokines, chemokines and related molecules in BCC. Studies thus far show that the factors described in this chapter play an integral role in BCC development and immunosuppression. A better understanding of these interactions may facilitate development of more potent immune-based treatment for BCC.

11. References

[1] Miller SJ. Biology of basal cell carcinoma (Part II). J Am Acad Dermatol 1991;24:161-175.
[2] Kaporis HG, Guttman-Yassky E, Lowes MA, *et al.* Human basal cell carcinoma is associated with Foxp3+ T cells in a Th2 dominant microenvironment. J Invest Dermatol 2007;127:2391-2398.
[3] Tjiu JW, Chen JS, Shun CT, *et al.* Tumor-associated macrophage-induced invasion and angiogenesis of human basal cell carcinoma cells by cyclooxygenase-2 induction. J Invest Dermatol 2009;129:1016-1025.
[4] Neuner P, Urbanski A, Trautinger F, *et al.* Increased IL-6 production by monocytes and keratinocytes in patients with psoriasis. J Invest Dermatol 1991;97:27-33.
[5] Jee SH, Shen SC, Chiu HC, Tsai WL, Kuo ML. Overexpression of interleukin-6 in human basal cell carcinoma cell lines increases anti-apoptotic activity and tumorigenic potency. Oncogene 2001;20:198-208.
[6] Jee SH, Chiu HC, Tsai TF, *et al.* The phosphotidyl inositol 3-kinase/Akt signal pathway is involved in interleukin-6-mediated Mcl-1 upregulation and anti-apoptosis activity in basal cell carcinoma cells. J Invest Dermatol 2002;119:1121-1127.
[7] Jee SH, Chu CY, Chiu HC, *et al.* Interleukin-6 induced basic fibroblast growth factor-dependent angiogenesis in basal cell carcinoma cell line via JAK/STAT3 and PI3-kinase/Akt pathways. J Invest Dermatol 2004;123:1169-1175.
[8] Chu CY, Cha ST, Lin WC, *et al.* Stromal cell-derived factor-1α (SDF-1α/CXCL12)-enhanced angiogenesis of human basal cell carcinoma cells involves ERK1/2–NF-κB/interleukin-6 pathway. Carcinogenesis 2009;30:205-213.
[9] Yen HT, Chiang LC, Wen KH, *et al.* The expression of cytokines by an established basal cell carcinoma cell line (BCC-1/KMC) compared with cultured normal keratinocytes. Arch Dermatol Res 1996;288:157-161.
[10] Gambichler T, Skrygan M, Hyun J, *et al.* Cytokine mRNA expression in basal cell carcinoma. Arch Dermatol Res 2006;298:139-141.
[11] Wilkening S, Hemminki K, Rudnai P, *et al.* Case-control study in basal cell carcinoma of the skin: single nucleotide polymorphisms in three interleukin promoters pre-analysed in pooled DNA. Br J Dermatol 2006;155:1139-1144.
[12] Festa F, Kumar R, Sanyal S, *et al.* Basal cell carcinoma and variants in genes coding for immune response, DNA repair, folate and iron metabolism. Mutat Res 2005;574:105-111.
[13] Chen Q, Daniel V, Maher DW, Hersey P. Production of IL-10 by melanoma cells: examination of its role in immunosuppression mediated by melanoma. Int J Cancer 1994;56:755-760.
[14] Krüger-Krasagakes S, Krasagakis K, Garbe C, *et al.* Expression of interleukin 10 in human melanoma. Br J Cancer 1994;70:1182-1185.

[15] Gerlini G, Tun-Kyi A, Dudli C, *et al.* Metastatic melanoma secreted IL-10 down-regulates CD1 molecules on dendritic cells in metastatic tumor lesions. Am J Pathol 2004;165:1853-1863.

[16] Kim J, Modlin RL, Moy RL, *et al.* IL-10 production in cutaneous basal and squamous cell carcinomas. A mechanism for evading the local T cell immune response. J Immunol 1995;155:2240-2247.

[17] Kooy AJ, Prens EP, Van Heukelum A, *et al.* Interferon-gamma-induced ICAM-1 and CD40 expression, complete lack of HLA-DR and CD80 (B7.1), and inconsistent HLA-ABC expression in basal cell carcinoma: a possible role for interleukin-10? J Pathol 1999;187:351-357.

[18] Itakura E, Huang RR, Wen DR, *et al.* IL-10 expression by primary tumor cells correlates with melanoma progression from radial to vertical growth phase and development of metastatic competence. Mod Pathol 2011;24:801-809.

[19] Urosevic M, Maier T, Benninghoff B, *et al.* Mechanisms underlying imiquimod-induced regression of basal cell carcinoma in vivo. Arch Dermatol 2003;139:1325-1332.

[20] Fernandes H, Fernandes N, Bhattacharya S, *et al.* Molecular signatures linked with aggressive behavior in Basal cell carcinoma: a report of 6 cases. Am J Dermatopathol 2010;32:550-556.

[21] Chen GS, Yu HS, Lan CC, *et al.* CXC chemokine receptor CXCR4 expression enhances tumorigenesis and angiogenesis of basal cell carcinoma. Br J Dermatol 2006;154:910-918.

[22] Chu CY, Cha ST, Chang CC, *et al.* Involvement of matrix metalloproteinase-13 in stromal-cell-derived factor 1α-directed invasion of human basal cell carcinoma cells. Oncogene 2007;26:2491-2501.

[23] Lo BKK, Yu M, Zloty D, *et al.* CXCR3/ligands are significantly involved in the tumorigenesis of basal cell carcinomas. Am J Pathol 2010;176:2435-2446.

[24] Lo BKK, Jalili RB, Zloty D, *et al.* CXCR3 ligands promote expression of functional indoleamine 2,3-dioxygenase (IDO) in basal cell carcinoma keratinocytes. Br J Dermatol 2011:Epub.

[25] Szepietowski JC, Walker C, McKenna DB, Hunter JA, McKenzie RC. Leukaemia inhibitory factor and interleukin-8 expression in nonmelanoma skin cancers. Clin Exp Dermatol 2001;26:72-78.

[26] Pivarcsi A, Muller A, Hippe A, *et al.* Tumor immune escape by the loss of homeostatic chemokine expression. Proc Natl Acad Sci U S A 2007;104:19055-19060.

[27] Kooy AJ, Tank B, Vuzevski VD, van Joost T, Prens EP. Expression of interferon-gamma receptors and interferon-gamma-induced up-regulation of intercellular adhesion molecule-1 in basal cell carcinoma; decreased expression of IFN-γR and shedding of ICAM-1 as a means to escape immune surveillance. J Pathol 1998;184:169-176.

[28] Wong DA, Bishop GA, Lowes MA, *et al.* Cytokine profiles in spontaneously regressing basal cell carcinomas. Br J Dermatol 2000;143:91-98.

[29] Hunt MJ, Halliday GM, Weedon D, Cooke BE, Barnetson RS. Regression in basal cell carcinoma: an immunohistochemical analysis. Brit J Dermatol 1994;130:1-8.

[30] Geisse J, Caro I, Lindholm J, *et al.* Imiquimod 5% cream for the treatment of superficial basal cell carcinoma: results from two phase III, randomized, vehicle-controlled studies. J Am Acad Dermatol 2004;50:722-733.

[31] Beutner KR, Geisse JK, Helman D, *et al.* Therapeutic response of basal cell carcinoma to the immune response modifier imiquimod 5% cream. J Am Acad Dermatol 1999;41:1002-1007.

[32] Schulze HJ, Cribier B, Requena L, *et al.* Imiquimod 5% cream for the treatment of superficial basal cell carcinoma: results from a randomized vehicle-controlled phase III study in Europe. Br J Dermatol 2005;152:939-947.

[33] Barnetson RS, Satchell A, Zhuang L, Slade HB, Halliday GM. Imiquimod induced regression of clinically diagnosed superficial basal cell carcinoma is associated with early infiltration by CD4 T cells and dendritic cells. Clin Exp Dermatol 2004;29:639-643.

[34] Wenzel J, Uerlich M, Haller O, Bieber T, Tueting T. Enhanced type I interferon signaling and recruitment of chemokine receptor CXCR3-expressing lymphocytes into the skin following treatment with the TLR7-agonist imiquimod. J Cutan Pathol 2005;32:257-262.

[35] Filipowicz E, Adegboyega P, Sanchez RL, Gatalica Z. Expression of CD95 (Fas) in sun-exposed human skin and cutaneous carcinomas. Cancer 2002;94:814-819.

[36] Buechner SA, Wernli M, Harr T, *et al.* Regression of basal cell carcinoma by intralesional interferon-alpha treatment is mediated by CD95 (Apo-1/Fas)–CD95 ligand-induced suicide. J Clin Invest 1997;100:2691-2696.

[37] Ji J, Wernli M, Mielgo A, Buechner SA, Erb P. Fas-ligand gene silencing in basal cell carcinoma tissue with small interfering RNA. Gene Ther 2005;12:678-684.

[38] Gutierrez-Steil C, Wrone-Smith T, Sun X, *et al.* Sunlight-induced basal cell carcinoma tumor cells and ultraviolet-B-irradiated psoriatic plaques express Fas ligand (CD95L). J Clin Invest 1998;101:33-39.

[39] Lee SH, Jang JJ, Lee JY, *et al.* Fas ligand is expressed in normal skin and in some cutaneous malignancies. Br J Dermatol 1998;139:186-191.

5

Metastatic Basal Cell Carcinoma

Anthony Vu and Donald Jr. Laub
University of Vermont,
College of Medicine
USA

1. Introduction

Basal cell carcinoma (BCC) is the most common skin malignancy, accounting for up to 80% of all cancers arising from the epidermis.[1] The disease usually presents as a slow growing, non-healing raised lesion with rolled borders and telangiectasias. These cancers arise from cells lining the deepest layer of the epidermis. BCC affects approximately 1 million Americans each year, more than squamous cell carcinoma and melanoma combined.[2] It is most commonly diagnosed in older, fair skinned individuals from ages 40-60.[3] Large amounts of sun exposure and UV radiation are the most common cause of BCC. Other etiologies include arsenic and various genetic disorders such as Nevus Sebaceous of Jadassohn, Xeroderma Pigmentosum, Basal Cell Nevus syndrome, Bazex syndrome, and Rombo syndrome.

An overwhelming majority of BCCs occur on the face or ear, but other likely sites include the neck, scalp, and upper trunk. Classically, it clinically presents as a pearly, non-healing, papulonodular lesion with rolled borders and telangiectasias, with or without ulcerations. These lesions are typically slow growing, minimally invasive, and thus have a very favorable prognosis. Surgical excision has long been considered the gold standard of treatment.[4]

2. Incidence

Since non-melanoma skin cancers are not reported in most cancer registries, it is hard to determine the exact yearly incidence of BCC. In a study by Miller et al.,[5] the age-

---

[1]Rubin, AI., Chen, EH., & Ratner, D. (2005). Basal-Cell Carcinoma. *New England Journal of Medicine*, Vol. 353, No. 21, (November 2005), pp. 2262-2269.
[2]Basal Cell Carinoma. n.d. In: *Skin Cancer Foundation*, May 2011, Available from: http://www.skincancer.org/basal-cell-carcinoma.html
[3]Chuang, TY., Popescu, A., Su, WP., & Chute, CG. (1990). Basal cell carcinoma: a population-based incidence study in Rochester, Minnesota. *Journal of the American Academy of Dermatology*, Vol. 22, No. 3, (March 1990), pp. 413-417.
[4]Bader, RS. (March 2011). Basal Cell Carcinoma, In: *Medscape Reference*, April 2011, Available from: http://emedicine.medscape.com/article/276624-overview
[5]Miller, DL. & Weinstock, MA. (1994). Nonmelanoma skin cancer in the United States: incidence. *Journal of the American Academy of Dermatology*, Vol. 30, No. 5.1, (May 1994), pp. 774-778

standardized yearly rates in the United States have been estimated at up to 407 cases of BCC per 100,000 white men and 212 cases per 100,000 white women. The yearly incidence is estimated to range between 900,000 and 1,200,000 cases per year with the trend towards an increasing number of cases each year. The estimated lifetime risk of BCC in the white population is 33-39% in men and 23-28% in women. In a population study of people younger than 40 years, the incidence of BCC per 100,000 persons was 25.9 for women and 20.9 for men.[6]

While the lifetime risk of BCC is high, it is well known to physicians that metastasis is relatively rare.[4] Using the criteria proposed by Lattes and Kessler in 1951, studies have indexed a metastasis rate of 0.0028-0.5%.[7] The proposed criteria for the diagnosis of metastatic BCC include:

1. The primary tumor must arise in the skin and not the mucous membranes
2. Metastases must be demonstrated at a site distant to the primary and must not be related to simple extension.
3. Histologic similarity between the primary tumor and the metastasis must exist.
4. The metastases must not have squamous cell features.

In a study by Wadhera et al., the currently published rate of metastasis was found to be higher than the reported numbers seem to show.[8] Using an incidence of 1 million cases per year in the United States and a metastasis rate of 0.0028%, there should be at least 30 cases of metastatic basal cell carcinoma (MBCC) per year. They report that this number conflicts with the number of cases reported to date. Dating back to 1894, when Beadles reported the first case of MBCC in a 56-year-old male, there have been around 300 reported cases, or an average of 3 cases of MBCC per year over 100 years. This discrepancy supports the idea that the current estimation of the rate of metastasis is incorrect and reporting of this disease in all cancer registries would be of great benefit.

3. Risk factors

3.1 Clinical

Several studies have tried to elucidate the clinical risk factors for metastasis. It is thought that primary tumors in the head and neck region have a higher metastatic potential; up to 85% of primary BCCs that metastasize originate from these regions.[9] Primary tumors arising

---

[6]Christenson, L., Borrowman, T., Vachon, C., Tellefson, M., Otley, C., Weaver, A., & Roenigk, R. (2005). Incidence of basal cell and squamous cell carcinomas in a population younger than 40 years. *Journal of the American Medical Association*, Vol. 294, No. 6, (August 2005), pp. 681–690.

[7]Lattes, R., & Kesser, RW. (1951). Metastasizing basal-cell epithelioma of the skin - Report of two cases. *Cancer*, Vol. 4, No. 4, (July 1951), pp. 866-878.

[8]Wadhera, A., Fazio, M., Bricca, G., & Stanton, O. (2006). Metastatic basal cell carincoma: A case report and literature review. How accurate is our incidence data? *Dermatology Online Journal*, Vol. 12, No. 5, (September 2006), pp. 7.

[9]Malone, JP., Fedok, FG., Belchis, DA., & Maloney, ME. (2000). Basal cell carcinoma metastatic to the parotid: report of a new case and review of the literature. *Ear Nose & Throat Journal*, Vol. 79, No. 7, (July 2000), pp.511–515, 518–519.

from the face alone account for at least two-thirds of metastatic BCC.[10] This may be related to the high concentration of blood vessels and thin skin around these areas.[11]

Tumors with any of the following characteristics have been thought to be high risk for metastatic potential: long duration, location in the mid face or ear, diameter larger than 2cm, aggressive histological subtype, previous treatment, neglected, or history of radiation.[12] There is a 2% incidence of metastasis for tumors larger than 3cm in diameter. The incidence increases to 25% for tumors larger than 5cm in diameter and 50% for tumors larger than 10cm in diameter.[1] Increased of tissue invasion and extension of the tumor into adjacent anatomical structures also enhance metastatic potential.[1] The male to female ratio is about 2:1.[13] Immunosuppression and evidence of perineural spread or invasion of blood vessels have also been implicated as risk factors for metastasis.[14]

3.2 Histopathologic

While clinical risk factors remain the most widely studied, others have tried to elucidate histopathologic risk factors associated with MBCC. BCC is made up of 5 major histological subtypes which include nodular, superficial, micronodular, infiltrating, and morpheaform. While nodular is thought to be the most common subtype,[15] there is no evidence that supports a particular subtype predisposes to MBCC.[16]

The concept of stromal dependence for primary tumor survival was first proposed in 1953 by Pinkus.[17] Several years later, this concept has proven to be applicable to metastatic tumors as well.[18] In a study with nude mice, successful transplantation of tumors occurred

---

[10]Grimwood, RE., Glanz, SM., & Siegle, RJ. (1988). Transplantation of human basal cell carcinoma to C57/Balb/Cbg/bg-nu/nu (nude) mouse. *The Journal of Dermatologic Surgery and Oncology*, Vol. 14, No. 1, (January 1988), pp. 59-62.

[10]Snow, SN., Sahl, W., Lo, JS., Mohs, FE., Warner, T., Dekkinga, JA., & Feyzi, J. (1994). Metastatic basal cell carcinoma. Report of five cases. *Cancer*, Vol. 73, No. 2, (January 1994), pp. 328-335.

[11]Cotran, RS. (1961). Metastasizing basal cell carcinomas. *Cancer*, Vol. 14., No. 5, (September-October 1961), pp. 1036-1040.

[12]Randle, HW. (1996). Basal cell carcinoma. Identification and treatment of the high-risk patient. *Dermatologic Surgery*, Vol. 22, No. 3, (March 1996), pp. 255-261.

[13]von Domarus, H. & Stevens, PJ. (1984). Metastatic basal cell carcinoma. Report of five cases and review of 170 cases in the literature. *Journal of the American Academy of Dermatology*, Vol. 10, No. 6, (June 1984), pp.1043-1060.

[14]Robinson, JK. & Dahiya, M. (2003). Basal cell carcinoma with pulmonary and lymph node metastasis causing death. *Archives of Dermatology*, Vol. 139, No. 5, (May 2003), pp. 643-648.

[15]Sexton, M., Jones, DB., & Maloney ME. (1990). Histologic pattern analysis of basal cell carcinoma. Study of a series of 1039 consecutive neoplasms. *Journal of the American Academy of Dermatology*, Vol. 23, No. 6.1, (December 1990), pp. 1118-1126.

[16]Berlin, JM., Warner, MR., & Bailin, PL. (2002). Metastatic basal cell carcinoma presenting as unilateral axillary lymphadenopathy: report of a case and review of the literature. *Dermatologic Surgery*, Vol. 28, No. 11, (November 2002), pp. 1082-1084.

[17]Pinkus, H. (1953). Premalignant fibroepithelioma tumors of the skin. *Archives of Dermatology*, Vol. 67, No. 6, (June 1953), pp. 598-615.

[18]Van Scott, EJ. & Reinertson, RP. (1961). The modulating influence of the stromal environment on epithelial cells studied in human autotransplants. *The Journal of Investigative Dermatology*, Vol. 36, Issue 2, (February 1961), pp. 109-131.

when accompanied with its surrounding stroma.[19] Other studies have failed to achieve successful transplantation when the tumors' stroma was not included.[20] Stromal dependency thus implies that either metastatic tumor cells are required to carry along their stroma or develop ways to support independent stromal proliferation in order to survive in a new location - perhaps explaining the low rate of metastasis.[17]

3.3 Cellular

Cytogenic aberrations have also been described in MBCC. Chromosomal abnormalities, specifically Trisomy 6, originating in primary tumor cells have been implicated as a factor in giving BCC its metastatic potential. In a study by Nangia et al., Trisomy 6 was identified in metastatic tumors cells of all four cases reported.[21] In addition, all twenty cases of nonaggressive BCCs showed no tumor cells with Trisomy 6 abnormalities. Immunohistochemical markers such as p53, Ki-67, and Bcl-2 can be helpful in differentiating aggressive versus non-aggressive BCCs.[22,23] Unfortunately, they have not proven to be distinguishing factors between metastatic and non-metastatic BCCs.[24]

4. Staging

The American Joint Committee On Cancer (AJCC) staging manual groups non-melanoma, non-Merkel cell skin cancers, including BCC, along with over 80 different types of other tumors in the cutaneous Squamous Cell Carcinoma Staging System.[25] As a result, the applicability of these guidelines to any individual cancer may be impaired. It is argued that some cutaneous tumors such as BCC do not require the staging needed for cutaneous squamous cell carcinomas, because of the infrequency of metastasis.[26] Although full staging is unnecessary for the majority of BCCs, the identification of high-risk behaviors should indicate the need for more in depth evaluation and staging.

---

[20]Lyles, TW., Freeman, RG., & Knox, JM. (1960). Transplantation of basal cell epitheliomas. *The Journal of Investigative Dermatology*, Vol. 34, No. 6, (June 1960), pp. 353.

[21]Nangia, R., Sait, SN., Block, AW., & Zhang, PJ. (2001). Trisomy 6 in basal cell carcinomas correlates with metastatic potential. *Cancer*, Vol. 91, No. 10, (May 2001), pp. 1927-1932.

[22]Abdelsayed, RA., Guijarro-Rojas, M., Ibrahim, NA., & Sangueza, OP. (2000). Immunohistochemical evaluation of basal cell carcinoma and trichepithelioma using Bcl-2, Ki67, PCNA and P53. *Journal of Cutaneous Pathology*, Vol. 27, No. 4, (April 2000), pp. 169–175.

[23]Staibano, S., Lo Muzio, L., Pannone, G., Scalvenzi, M., Salvatore, G., Errico, ME., Fanali, S., De Rosa, G., & Piattelli, A. (2001). Interaction between bcl-2 and P53 in neoplastic progression of basal cell carcinoma of the head and neck. *Anticancer Research*, Vol. 21, No. 6A, (November-December 2001), pp. 3757–3764.

[24]Ionescu, DN., Arida, M., & Jukic, DM. (2006). Metastatic basal cell carcinoma: four case reports, review of literature, and immunohistochemical evaluation. *Archives of Pathology and Laboratory Medicine*, Vol. 130, No. 1, (January 2006), pp. 45-51.

[25]Edge, SE., Byrd, DR., Compton, CC., Fritz, AG., Greene, FL., & Trotti, A., (Ed(s).). (2009) *American Joint Committee On Cancer: Cancer Staging Manual, 7th edition*, Springer, 978-0-387-88440-0, New York, NY, USA.

[26]Warner, CL & Cockerell, CJ. (2011). The new 7th edition American Joint Committee On Cancer staging of cutaneous non-melanoma skin cancer: a critical review. *American Journal of Clinical Dermatology*, Vol. 12, No. 3, (June 2011), pp. 147-154.

Based on current research, depth of invasion may be the most important tumor variable associated with prognosis (See Table 1). In a study by Rowe et al., the presence of either tumor thickness >4mm or depth of invasion ≥Clark level IV was found to be associated with an increased risk of recurrence by a factor of 2, as well as an increase in the risk of metastasis by a factor of 5.[27] Similar to melanoma, there is evidence that Breslow thickness may be more important for determining prognosis in non-melanoma cutaneous carcinoma than Clark's level, although both are predictive of advanced disease. Additionally, while early studies identified Breslow thickness >4mm as predictive of aggressive behavior, subsequent studies have shown that a 2mm cutoff more appropriately stratifies low and high-risk lesions.[26]

Primary tumor (T)*.

Tx	Primary tumor cannot be assessed
T0	No evidence of primary tumor
Tis	Carcinoma in situ
T1	Carcinoma less than 2cm in greatest dimension, with less than 2 high risk features**
T2	Carcinoma greater than 2cm in greatest dimension, Or Tumor of any size with at least 2 high risk features**
T3	Tumor invasion of the maxilla, mandible, orbit, or temporal bone
T4	Tumor invasion of the skeleton (appendicular or axial) or with perineural involvement of the skull base

*Excludes cutaneous squamous cell carcinoma of the eyelid.
**High-risk features for the primary tumor (T) staging: Depth/invasion: >2mm thickness, Clark level ≥IV, Perineural invasion. Anatomic location: Primary site ear, Primary site non-hair-bearing lip. Differentiation: Poorly differentiated or undifferentiated. From the American Joint Committee On Cancer 7th edition "Cutaneous Squamous Cell Carcinoma and Other Cutaneous Carcinomas."

Table 1. Primary Tumor (T) Staging.

Perineural invasion has also been found to be a significant indicator of high-risk disease.[1,28] Although less commonly identified (only present in 5 percent of non-melanoma cutaneous carcinomas), there is some evidence that perineural invasion is associated with an increase in both the recurrence rate and the metastatic rate by a factor of 5.[27] As perineural spread can be difficult to follow histologically and clinically, such tumors can spread much more prior to detection. The diagnosis of perineural invasion carries a generally dismal prognosis, as the 5-year mortality rate approaches 90%.[28]

The 7th edition AJCC manual chose to include advanced tumor depth/invasion (defined as >2mm in thickness, ≥Clark level IV) among the high-risk features capable of upstaging a T1 neoplasm. Overall, this represents an improvement over previous editions, as it allows for

[27]Rowe, DE., Carroll, RJ., & Day, CL Jr. (1992). Prognostic factors for local recurrence, metastasis, and survival rates in squamous cell carcinoma of the skin, ear, and lip. Implications for treatment modality selection. *Journal of the American Academy of Dermatology*, Vol. 26, No. 6, (June 1992), pp. 976-990.

[28]Garcia-Serra, A., Hinerman, RW., Mendenhall, WM., Amdur, RJ., Morris, CG., Williams, LS., & Mancuso, AA. (2003). Carcinoma of the skin with perineural invasion. *Head & Neck*, Vol. 25, No. 12, (December 2003), pp. 1027-1033.

the identification of a subset of lesions that, although small in size, nevertheless are likely to demonstrate aggressive clinical behavior.[29,30]

The final high-risk feature identified in the 7th edition of the AJCC: Cancer Staging Manual guidelines is the location of the primary tumor on high-risk anatomic sites. This is based on evidence that lesions located on the lip and ear are more aggressive compared to tumors presenting on other locations throughout the body.[31] These anatomic sites are associated with recurrence and metastatic rates between 10 to 25 percent. Similar to the previously mentioned high-risk variants, recognition of the increased risk associated with these sites. Warner and Cockerell feel that tumors located on the central face and dorsal hands and feet also should be considered high-risk sites.[26]

Recurrent disease is a high-risk factor worth special discussion. Recurrent or persistent diseases are strong prognostic factors for metastasis.[3,32] Recurrent or previously treated tumors tend to be more aggressive, less responsive to treatment, and associated with decreased survival (78% 5-year survival compared to 97% for primary lesions).[33] Although rarely performed for Non-Melanoma Cutaneous Carcinoma, the current TNM staging system, denotes recurrent neoplasms with an "r" qualifier prior to TNM-specific designations For example, a locally recurrent tumor greater than 2cm in size, without evidence of lymph node involvement or metastasis would be staged as: rT2N0M0. As a result, a subset of high-risk lesions is clearly defined as such, and data collection for these tumors can be significantly enhanced. T3 tumors are now classified as those with bony extension to the mandible, maxilla, temple, or orbit whereas the T4 designation is reserved for perineural involvement of the skull base or bony extension to the axial or appendicular skeleton.

Under the 7th edition of the AJCC Cancer Staging Manual guidelines (See table 2), metastasis to a single node less than 3cm in greatest dimension is defined as N1. The N2 designation refers to either a single node 3–6cm in size, or multinodal disease where no individual node is greater than 6cm in size. Based on the specific pattern of nodal involvement, N2 is subcategorized into three separate groupings. Involvement of a single ipsilateral node is categorized as N2a, metastasis to multiple ipsilateral nodes as N2b, and involvement of contralateral or bilateral lymph nodes as N2c. The N3 designation is reserved for any lymph node greater than 6cm in greatest dimension, regardless of number of nodes involved.

---

[29]Lardaro, T., Shea, SM., Sarfman, W., Liegeois, N., & Sober, AJ. (2010). Improvements in the staging of cutaneous squamous-cell carcinoma in the 7th edition of the American Joint Committee On Cancer: Cancer Staging Manual. *Annals of Surgical Oncology*, Vol. 17, No. 8, (August 2010), pp. 1979–1980.

[30]Buethe, D., Warner, C., Miedler, J., & Cockerell, CJ. (2011). Focus Issue on Squamous Cell Carcinoma: Practical Concerns Regarding the 7th Edition American Joint Committee On Cancer: Staging Guidelines. *Journal of Skin Cancer*, Vol. 2011, Article ID 156391, (2011), 9 pages.

[31]Preston, DS. & Stern, RS. (1992). Nonmelanoma cancers of the skin. *The New England Journal of Medicine*, Vol. 327, No. 23, (December 1992), pp. 1649-1662.

[32]Rowe, DE., Carroll, RJ., & Day, CL Jr. (1992). Prognostic factors for local recurrence, metastasis, and survival rates in squamous cell carcinoma of the skin, ear, and lip. Implications for treatment modality selection. *Journal of the American Academy of Dermatology*, Vol. 26, No. 6, (June 1992), pp. 976-990.

[33]Andruchow, JL., Veness, MJ., Morgan, GJ., Gao, K., Clifford, A., Shannon, KF., Poulsen, M., Kenny, L., Palme, CE., Gullane, P., Morris, C., Mendenhall, WM., Patel, KN., Shah, JP., & O'Brien, CJ. (2006). Implications for clinical staging of metastatic cutaneous squamous carcinoma of the head and neck based on a multicenter study of treatment outcomes. *Cancer*, Vol. 106, No. 5, (March 2006), pp. 1078-1083.

The distant metastasis designation of the 7th edition of the AJCC Cutaneous Squamous Cell Carcinoma staging system is unchanged from previous editions (See table 3). Importantly, there is no provision for classification of lymph node metastasis far removed from regional nodal basins as distant metastasis.[26]

Regional lymph nodes (N).

Nx	Regional lymph nodes cannot be assessed.
N0	No regional lymph node metastases.
N1	Metastasis in a single ipsilateral lymph node, 3cm or less in greatest dimension.
N2	Metastasis in a single ipsilateral lymph node, more than 3cm but not more than 6cm in greatest dimension; or in multiple ipsilateral lymphnodes, none more than 6cm in greatest dimension; or in bilateral or contralateral lymph nodes, none more than 6cm in greatest dimension.
N2a	Metastasis in a single ipsilateral lymph node, more than 3cm but not more than 6cm in greatest dimension.
N2b	Metastasis in multiple ipsilateral lymph nodes, none more than 6cm in greatest dimension.
N2c	Metastasis in bilateral or contralateral lymph nodes, none more than 6cm in greatest dimension.
N3	Metastasis in a lymph node, more than 6cm in greatest dimension.

Table 2. Regional Lymph Node (N) Staging.

Distant metastasis (M).

M0	No distant metastasis
M1	Distant metastasis

Table 3. Metastasis (M) Staging.

The staging groups offer reasonable stratification of patients based on prognosis (See table 4). Briefly, T1 and T2 tumors are assigned Stage I and Stage II, respectively, Stage III includes all T3 or N1 tumors that do not meet criteria for Stage IV, and the presence of any T4, N2-3, or M1 designation is required for Stage IV classification.[27]

Anatomic stage/prognostic groups.

Stage 0	Tis	N0	M0
Stage I	T1	N0	M0
Stage II	T2	N0	M0
Stage III	T3	N0	M0
	T1	N1	M0
	T2	N1	M0
	T3	N1	M0
Stage IV	T1	N2	M0
	T2	N2	M0
	T3	N2	M0
	T Any	N3	M0
	T4	N Any	M0
	T Any	N Any	M1

Table 4. Staging Classification.

Cutaneous neoplasms that rarely metastasize, such as BCC, full staging is often unnecessary and perhaps should be mentioned in the staging guidelines as an exception.[33] In other cases, although relevant, full initial evaluation of high-risk features may not be possible, as primary biopsies frequently involve only a small portion of the primary tumor, precluding accurate assessment. Moreover, surgeons and dermatologists need to alter their clinical practice and begin assessing for vertical depth of invasion. Other issues that need to be clarified include the definition of tumors of the lip and the histologic designation of "poorly differentiated" and "undifferentiated" neoplasms.[30] However, the incorporation of these factors might be impractical for widespread use in clinical practice.[1]

There is a single report of the use of sentinel lymph node biopsy in high-risk lesions.[34] This approach would not detect any hematogenous spread, and so its role in the staging of the disease remains to be determined.

5. Treatment

Treatment for non-MBCC can be either surgical or nonsurgical. Surgical excision is generally curative with five-year cure rates of more than 99 percent for primary tumors not involving the head.[35] For lesions involving the head, the five-year cure rate is 97 percent for lesions less than 6mm and 92 percent for lesions greater than 6mm. Other surgical options include Mohs micrographic surgery, curettage and electrodessication, and cryosurgery. In a Cochrane review of different treatment modalities, one study showed no significant difference between Mohs micrographic surgery and surgical excision in recurrence rates at 30 months for high-risk facial BCCs.[36]

Non-surgical options include radiotherapy, photodynamic therapy, and topical therapy. In one randomized control trial of surgery versus radiotherapy, surgery provided significantly better cure rates when compared to radiotherapy. [36] Radiotherapy has been shown to provide better cure rates when compared to cryosurgery. Imiquimod cream has shown promising early results but long-term data is lacking.[36] With un-reviewed information available on the Internet and an un-regulated herbal therapeutic industry, patients will self-treat tumors with anecdotally supported alternative medicine.[37] We discourage the use of these forms of treatment, especially within the current culture of practicing evidence-based medicine.[38]

There are currently no established guidelines for the treatment of metastatic disease specifically because all forms of treatment thus far have provided dismal results in terms of morbidity and mortality. Primary BCC metastasizes usually via lymphatics, although it can also spread hematogenously. Metastasis most commonly occurs in regional lymph nodes,

---

[34]Harwood M, Wu H, Tanabe K, et al. Metastatic basal cell carcinoma diagnosed by sentinel lymph node biopsy. J Am Acad Dermatol 2005; 3:475-8.

[35]Silverman, MK., Kopf, AW., Bart, RS., Grin, CM., & Levenstein, MS. (1992). Recurrence rates of treated basal cell carcinomas. Part 3: surgical excision. *The Journal of Dermatologic Surgery and Oncology*, Vol. 18, No. 6, (June 1992), pp. 471-476.

[36]Bath-Hextall, FJ., Perkins, W., Bong, J., & Williams, HC. (2007). Interventions for basal cell carcinoma of the skin, In: *Cochrane Database of Systematic Reviews*, Issue 1, (January 2007), Art. No.: CD003412.

[37]Laub, DR Jr. (2008). Death from metastatic basal cell carcinoma: herbal remedy or just unlucky? *Journal of Plastic, Reconstructive, & Aesthetic Surgery*, Vol. 61, No. 7, (July 2008), pp. 846-848.

[38]McDaniel S, Goldman GD (2002) Consequences of using escharotic agents as primary treatment for nonmelanoma skin cancer. *Archives of Dermatol*ogy Vol. 138, No.12, (December 2002), pp. 1593-6.

lung, and bone although there have been documented cases involving the spinal cord, parotid gland, skin, bone marrow, spleen, liver, adrenal glands, brain, dura mater, esophagus, heart, and kidney. The prognosis for these patients is poor with a mean survival time of only 8 months from the time at diagnosis.[5] In cases where metastasis is only to lymph nodes, patients live up to an average of 3.6 years.[39] There has been one reported case in which a patient lived 25 years after diagnosis.[40] Median age at the first sign of metastasis is 59 years while the median interval between the onset of the primary tumor and the first sign of metastasis is 9 years.[13] Systemic chemotherapy has been attempted with mixed results. Combinations of 5-fluorouracil, bleomycin, and methotrexate have been unsuccessful.[41,42] However, there has been one case with a positive response to cyclophosphamide and cis-diamine dichloroplatinum in a patient with pulmonary metastasis.[43] Cisplatin-based therapy has also been shown to be of benefit for patients with metastasis.[44,45]

Surgical resection is recommended for isolated metastasis, as the results of systemic chemotheraputic treatment are generally not as promising. Ducic and Mara treated metastatic lesions to the parotid gland with parotidectomy with adjuvant radiation therapy with good results.[46] Presentation with widely disseminated disease would not allow this approach, however.

It has long been thought that treatment of primary cancers with radiotherapy can contribute to their metastatic potential, although there is no evidence to support this. In fact, the incidence of MBCC in patients treated primarily by radiotherapy is estimated to be 1 in 25,000, which is much less than the incidence of MBCC in all patients with primary tumors.[47] There have been, however, case reports in which radiotherapy has been found to be beneficial in the treatment of metastatic disease.[48] In cases where clear surgical margins

---

[39]Raszewski, RL. & Guyuron, B. (1990). Long-term survival following nodal metastases from basal cell carcinoma. *Annals of Plastic Surgery*, Vol. 24, No. 2, (February 1990), pp. 170-175.

[40]Lo, JS., Snow, SN., Reizner, GT., Mohs, FE., Larson, PO., & Hruza GJ. (1991). Metastatic basal cell carcinoma: report of twelve cases with a review of the literature. *Journal of the American Academy of Dermatology*, Vol. 24, No. 5.1, (May 1991), pp. 715-719.

[41]Costanza, ME., Dayal, Y., Binder, S., Nathanson, L., Safai, B., & Good R.A. (1974). Metastatic basal cell carcinoma: Review, report of a case and chemotherapy. *Cancer*, Vol. 34, No. 1, (July 1974), pp. 230-235.

[42]Bason, MM., Grant-Kels, JM., & Govil, CT. Metastatic basal cell carcinoma: response to chemotherapy. *Journal of the American Academy of Dermatology*, Vol. 22, No. 5, (May 1990), pp. 905-908.

[43]Woods, RL. & Steward, JF. (1980). Metastatic basal cell carcinoma: report of a case responding to chemotherapy. *Postgraduate Medical Journal*, Vol. 56, No. 654, (May 1980), pp. 272-273.

[44]Khandekar, J. (1990). Complete response of metastatic basal cell carcinoma to cisplatin chemotherapy: A report on two patients. *Archives of Dermatology*, Vol. 126, No. 12, (December 1990), pp. 1660.

[45]Moeholt, K., Aagaard, H., Pfeiffer, P., & Hansen, O. (1996). Platinum-based cytotoxic therapy in basal cell carcinoma – a review of the literature. *Acta Oncologica*, Vol. 35, No. 6, (January 1996), pp. 677–682.

[46]Ducic Y, Marra DE. Metastatic basal cell carcinoma Am J Otolaryngol. [Epub ahead of print] (October 2010)

[47]Christie, D. The benefit of radiotherapy in metastatic basal cell carcinoma. *Australian and New Zealand Journal of Surgery*, (July 1997), Vol. 67, No. 7, pp. 491–493.

[48]Ozgediz, D., Smith, EB., Zheng, J., Otero, J., Tabatabai, Z., & Corvera, C. (2008). Basal cell carcinoma does metastasize. *Dermatology Online Journal*, Vol. 14, No. 8, August 2008, Article 5.
Available at: http://dermatology-s10.cdlib.org/148/case_reports/bcc/corvera.html

may be difficult to obtain, radiotherapy can offer an advantage of tissue preservation in patients with large lesions through deep tissue penetration.

More recently, a clinical trial with GDC-0449, a small-molecule inhibitor of smoothened homologue (SMO), has shown promising results. SMO is involved in activation of the hedgehog pathway that has been implicated in the development of BCC[49] and various other cancers.[50] In a phase 1 trial by Von Hoff et al., GDC-0449 was used to treat 33 patients with locally advanced or MBCC.[51] Of the 15 patients with locally advanced disease, 60% of patients showed a good response. Of the 18 patients with metastatic disease, 50% of patients showed a good response.

The management of patients with suspected metastasis often involves obtaining a CT or MRI scan to look for evidence of occult disease. Recently, a study using FDG-PET has proven to be effective in detecting subclinical disease in a man presenting with multiple primary cutaneous lesions.[52] While further studies are required, FDG PET may prove to be more effective than both CT and MRI in the radiographic evaluation of suspected metastatic disease.

6. Conclusion

BCC generally follows a very predictable clinical course from the time of diagnosis to subsequent treatment. The standard of care is surgical excision, which provides excellent cure rates. Other methods of treatment include radiotherapy, photodynamic therapy, cryotherapy and topical chemotherapy.

For patients with metastatic disease, morbidity and mortality remains exceedingly high. The biggest risk factors for metastasis are tumor size, depth, and recurrence. Primary tumors arising from the mid face and ears provide a majority of the cases of metastasis but this is also the case for non-metastasizing BCC.

With the exception of platinum-based chemotherapeutic agents, combinations of most other forms of chemotherapy with radiation and/or surgery have not improved mortality rates. It is clear that the development of metastatic potential in BCC, like many cancers, is multi-factorial in etiology. Research aimed at the clinical, histopathologic, and molecular characteristics of metastasis has helped us better understand the risk factors associated with such rare occurrences. As we further our understanding of the pathogenesis behind MBCC, more promising drugs such as GDC-0449 will be developed.

---

[49]Johnson, R., Rothman, A., Xie, J., Goodrich, L., Bare, J., Bonifas, J., Quinn, A., Myers, R., Cox, D., Epstein, E., & Scott M. (1996). Human homolog of patched, a candidate gene for the basal cell nevus syndrome. *Science*, Vol. 272, No. 5268, (June 1996), pp. 1668-1671.

[50]Katoh, Y. & Katoh, M. (2009). Hedgehog target genes: mechanisms of carcinogenesis induced by aberrant hedgehog signaling activation. *Current Molecular Medicine*, Vol. 9, No. 7, (September 2009), pp. 873-886.

[51]Von Hoff, D., LoRusso, PM., Rudin, CM., Reddy, JC., Yauch, RL., Tibes, R., Weiss, GJ., Borad, MJ., Hann, CL., Brahmer, JR., Mackey, HM., Lum, BL., Darbonne, WC., Marsters, JC Jr., de Sauvage, FJ., & Low, JA. (2009). Inhibition of the Hedgehog Pathway in Advanced Basal-Cell Carcinoma. *The New England Journal of Medicine*, Vol. 361, No. 12, (September 2009), pp. 1164-1172.

[52]Niederkohr, RD. & Gamie, SH. (2007). F-18 FDG PET as an imaging tool for detecting and staging metastatic basal-cell carcinoma. *Clinical Nuclear Medicine*, Vol. 32, No. 6, (June 2007), pp. 491-492.

The incidence of BCC will continue to increase over the years as the baby-boomer generation continues to age. Although the estimated rates of metastasis are low, there will still be a growing number of patients that will need treatment for this presently incurable disease. Physicians need to be aware of the poor prognosis that MBCC carries. Because adequate treatments are not available for metastasis, prevention should be practiced by all providers through vigilant monitoring of suspicious skin lesions and early surgical excision of primary tumor.

7. References

Abdelsayed, RA., Guijarro-Rojas, M., Ibrahim, NA., & Sangueza, OP. (2000). Immunohistochemical evaluation of basal cell carcinoma and trichepithelioma using Bcl-2, Ki67, PCNA and P53. *Journal of Cutaneous Pathology*, Vol. 27, No. 4, (April 2000), pp. 169–175.

Andruchow, JL., Veness, MJ., Morgan, GJ., Gao, K., Clifford, A., Shannon, KF., Poulsen, M., Kenny, L., Palme, CE., Gullane, P., Morris, C., Mendenhall, WM., Patel, KN., Shah, JP., & O'Brien, CJ. (2006). Implications for clinical staging of metastatic cutaneous squamous carcinoma of the head and neck based on a multicenter study of treatment outcomes. *Cancer*, Vol. 106, No. 5, (March 2006), pp. 1078-1083.

Bader, RS. (March 2011). Basal Cell Carcinoma, In: *Medscape Reference*, April 2011, Available from: http://emedicine.medscape.com/article/276624-overview

Basal Cell Carinoma. n.d. In: *Skin Cancer Foundation*, May 2011, Available from: http://www.skincancer.org/basal-cell-carcinoma.html

Bason, MM., Grant-Kels, JM., & Govil, CT. Metastatic basal cell carcinoma: response to chemotherapy. *Journal of the American Academy of Dermatology*, Vol. 22, No. 5, (May 1990), pp. 905-908.

Bath-Hextall, FJ., Perkins, W., Bong, J., & Williams, HC. (2007). Interventions for basal cell carcinoma of the skin, In: *Cochrane Database of Systematic Reviews*, Issue 1, (January 2007), Art. No.: CD003412.

Berlin, JM., Warner, MR., & Bailin, PL. (2002). Metastatic basal cell carcinoma presenting as unilateral axillary lymphadenopathy: report of a case and review of the literature. *Dermatologic Surgery*, Vol. 28, No. 11, (November 2002), pp. 1082-1084.

Buethe, D., Warner, C., Miedler, J., & Cockerell, CJ. (2011). Focus Issue on Squamous Cell Carcinoma: Practical Concerns Regarding the 7th Edition American Joint Committee On Cancer: Staging Guidelines. *Journal of Skin Cancer*, Vol. 2011, Article ID 156391, (2011), 9 pages.

Christenson, L., Borrowman, T., Vachon, C., Tellefson, M., Otley, C., Weaver, A., & Roenigk, R. (2005). Incidence of basal cell and squamous cell carcinomas in a population younger than 40 years. *Journal of the American Medical Association*, Vol. 294, No. 6, (August 2005), pp. 681–690.

Christie, D. The benefit of radiotherapy in metastatic basal cell carcinoma. *Australian and New Zealand Journal of Surgery*, (July 1997), Vol. 67, No. 7, pp. 491–493.

Chuang, TY., Popescu, A., Su, WP., & Chute, CG. (1990). Basal cell carcinoma: a population-based incidence study in Rochester, Minnesota. *Journal of the American Academy of Dermatology*, Vol. 22, No. 3, (March 1990), pp. 413-417.

Costanza, ME., Dayal, Y., Binder, S., Nathanson, L., Safai, B., & Good R.A. (1974). Metastatic basal cell carcinoma: Review, report of a case and chemotherapy. *Cancer*, Vol. 34, No. 1, (July 1974), pp. 230-235.

Cotran, RS. (1961). Metastasizing basal cell carcinomas. *Cancer*, Vol. 14., No. 5, (September-October 1961), pp. 1036-1040.

Ducic Y. & Marra DE. (2010) Metastatic basal cell carcinoma *American Journal of Otolaryngology* [Epub ahead of print] (October 2010)

Edge, SE., Byrd, DR., Compton, CC., Fritz, AG., Greene, FL., & Trotti, A., (Ed(s).). (2009) *American Joint Committee on Cancer: Cancer Staging Manual, 7th edition*, Springer, 978-0-387-88440-0, New York, NY, USA.

Garcia-Serra, A., Hinerman, RW., Mendenhall, WM., Amdur, RJ., Morris, CG., Williams, LS., & Mancuso, AA. (2003). Carcinoma of the skin with perineural invasion. *Head & Neck*, Vol. 25, No. 12, (December 2003), pp. 1027-1033.

Grimwood, RE., Glanz, SM., & Siegle, RJ. (1988). Transplantation of human basal cell carcinoma to C57/Balb/Cbg/bg-nu/nu (nude) mouse. *The Journal of Dermatologic Surgery and Oncology*, Vol. 14, No. 1, (January 1988), pp. 59-62.

Harwood M, Wu H, Tanabe K & Bercovitch L. (2005). Metastatic basal cell carcinoma diagnosed by sentinel lymph node biopsy. *Journal of the American Academy of Dermatology* Vol. 53, No. 3, (September 2005), pp. 475-8.

Ionescu, DN., Arida, M., & Jukic, DM. (2006). Metastatic basal cell carcinoma: four case reports, review of literature, and immunohistochemical evaluation. Archives of *Pathology and Laboratory Medicine*, Vol. 130, No. 1, (January 2006), pp. 45-51.

Johnson, R., Rothman, A., Xie, J., Goodrich, L., Bare, J., Bonifas, J., Quinn, A., Myers, R., Cox, D., Epstein, E., & Scott M. (1996). Human homolog of patched, a candidate gene for the basal cell nevus syndrome. Science, Vol. 272, No. 5268, (June 1996), pp. 1668-1671.

Katoh, Y. & Katoh, M. (2009). Hedgehog target genes: mechanisms of carcinogenesis induced by aberrant hedgehog signaling activation. *Current Molecular Medicine*, Vol. 9, No. 7, (September 2009), pp. 873-886.

Khandekar, J. (1990). Complete response of metastatic basal cell carcinoma to cisplatin chemotherapy: A report on two patients. *Archives of Dermatology*, Vol. 126, No. 12, (December 1990), pp. 1660.

Lardaro, T., Shea, SM., Sarfman, W., Liegeois, N., & Sober, AJ. (2010). Improvements in the staging of cutaneous squamous-cell carcinoma in the 7th edition of the American Joint Committee On Cancer: Cancer Staging Manual. *Annals of Surgical Oncology*, Vol. 17, No. 8, (August 2010), pp. 1979–1980.

Lattes, R., & Kesser, RW. (1951). Metastasizing basal-cell epithelioma of the skin - Report of two cases. *Cancer*, Vol. 4, No. 4, (July 1951), pp. 866-878.

Laub, DR Jr. (2008). Death from metastatic basal cell carcinoma: herbal remedy or just unlucky? *Journal of Plastic, Reconstructive, & Aesthetic Surgery*, Vol. 61, No. 7, (July 2008), pp. 846-848.

Lo, JS., Snow, SN., Reizner, GT., Mohs, FE., Larson, PO., & Hruza GJ. (1991). Metastatic basal cell carcinoma: report of twelve cases with a review of the literature. *Journal of the American Academy of Dermatology*, Vol. 24, No. 5.1, (May 1991), pp. 715-719.

Lyles, TW., Freeman, RG., & Knox, JM. (1960). Transplantation of basal cell epitheliomas. *The Journal of Investigative Dermatology*, Vol. 34, No. 6, (June 1960), pp. 353.

Malone, JP., Fedok, FG., Belchis, DA., & Maloney, ME. (2000). Basal cell carcinoma metastatic to the parotid: report of a new case and review of the literature. *Ear Nose & Throat Journal*, Vol. 79, No. 7, (July 2000), pp.511–515, 518–519.

McDaniel S & Goldman GD (2002) Consequences of using escharotic agents as primary treatment for nonmelanoma skin cancer. *Archives of Dermatology* Vol. 138, No.12, (December 2002), pp. 1593-6.

Miller, DL. & Weinstock, MA. (1994). Nonmelanoma skin cancer in the United States: incidence. *Journal of the American Academy of Dermatology*, Vol. 30, No. 5.1, (May 1994), pp. 774-778.

Moeholt, K., Aagaard, H., Pfeiffer, P., & Hansen, O. (1996). Platinum-based cytotoxic therapy in basal cell carcinoma – a review of the literature. *Acta Oncologica*, Vol. 35, No. 6, (January 1996), pp. 677–682.

Nangia, R., Sait, SN., Block, AW., & Zhang, PJ. (2001). Trisomy 6 in basal cell carcinomas correlates with metastatic potential. *Cancer*, Vol. 91, No. 10, (May 2001), pp. 1927-1932.

Niederkohr, RD. & Gamie, SH. (2007). F-18 FDG PET as an imaging tool for detecting and staging metastatic basal-cell carcinoma. *Clinical Nuclear Medicine*, Vol. 32, No. 6, (June 2007), pp. 491-492.

Ozgediz, D., Smith, EB., Zheng, J., Otero, J., Tabatabai, Z., & Corvera, C. (2008). Basal cell carcinoma does metastasize. *Dermatology Online Journal*, Vol. 14, No. 8, August 2008, Article 5. Available at:
http://dermatology-s10.cdlib.org/148/case_reports/bcc/corvera.html

Pinkus, H. (1953). Premalignant fibroepithelioma tumors of the skin. *Archives of Dermatology*, Vol. 67, No. 6, (June 1953), pp. 598-615.

Preston, DS. & Stern, RS. (1992). Nonmelanoma cancers of the skin. *The New England Journal of Medicine*, Vol. 327, No. 23, (December 1992), pp. 1649-1662.

Quaedvlieg, PJ., Creytens, DH., Epping, GG., Peutz-Kootstra, CJ., Nieman, FH., Thissen, MR., & Krekels, GA. (2006). Histopathological characteristics of metastasizing squamous cell carcinoma of the skin and lips. *Histopathology*, Vol. 49, No. 3, (September 2006), pp. 256-264.

Randle, HW. (1996). Basal cell carcinoma. Identification and treatment of the high-risk patient. *Dermatologic Surgery*, Vol. 22, No. 3, (March 1996), pp. 255-261.

Raszewski, RL. & Guyuron, B. (1990). Long-term survival following nodal metastases from basal cell carcinoma. *Annals of Plastic Surgery*, Vol. 24, No. 2, (February 1990), pp. 170-175.

Robinson, JK. & Dahiya, M. (2003). Basal cell carcinoma with pulmonary and lymph node metastasis causing death. *Archives of Dermatology*, Vol. 139, No. 5, (May 2003), pp. 643-648.

Rowe, DE., Carroll, RJ., & Day, CL Jr. (1992). Prognostic factors for local recurrence, metastasis, and survival rates in squamous cell carcinoma of the skin, ear, and lip. Implications for treatment modality selection. *Journal of the American Academy of Dermatology*, Vol. 26, No. 6, (June 1992), pp. 976-990.

Rubin, AI., Chen, EH., & Ratner, D. (2005). Basal-Cell Carcinoma. *New England Journal of Medicine*, Vol. 353, No. 21, (November 2005), pp. 2262-2269.

Sexton, M., Jones, DB., & Maloney ME. (1990). Histologic pattern analysis of basal cell carcinoma. Study of a series of 1039 consecutive neoplasms. *Journal of the American Academy of Dermatology*, Vol. 23, No. 6.1, (December 1990), pp. 1118-1126.

Silverman, MK., Kopf, AW., Bart, RS., Grin, CM., & Levenstein, MS. (1992). Recurrence rates of treated basal cell carcinomas. Part 3: surgical excision. *The Journal of Dermatologic Surgery and Oncology*, Vol. 18, No. 6, (June 1992), pp. 471-476.

Snow, SN., Sahl, W., Lo, JS., Mohs, FE., Warner, T., Dekkinga, JA., & Feyzi, J. (1994). Metastatic basal cell carcinoma. Report of five cases. *Cancer*, Vol. 73, No. 2, (January 1994), pp. 328-335.

Staibano, S., Lo Muzio, L., Pannone, G., Scalvenzi, M., Salvatore, G., Errico, ME., Fanali, S., De Rosa, G., & Piattelli, A. (2001). Interaction between bcl-2 and P53 in neoplastic progression of basal cell carcinoma of the head and neck. *Anticancer Research*, Vol. 21, No. 6A, (November-December 2001), pp. 3757–3764.

Van Scott, EJ. & Reinertson, RP. (1961). The modulating influence of the stromal environment on epithelial cells studied in human autotransplants. *The Journal of Investigative Dermatology*, Vol. 36, Issue 2, (February 1961), pp. 109-131.

von Domarus, H. & Stevens, PJ., (1984). Metastatic basal cell carcinoma. Report of five cases and review of 170 cases in the literature. *Journal of the American Academy of Dermatology*, Vol. 10, No. 6, (June 1984), pp.1043-1060.

Von Hoff, D., LoRusso, PM., Rudin, CM., Reddy, JC., Yauch, RL., Tibes, R., Weiss, GJ., Borad, MJ., Hann, CL., Brahmer, JR., Mackey, HM., Lum, BL., Darbonne, WC., Marsters, JC Jr., de Sauvage, FJ., & Low, JA. (2009). Inhibition of the Hedgehog Pathway in Advanced Basal-Cell Carcinoma. *The New England Journal of Medicine*, Vol. 361, No. 12, (September 2009), pp. 1164-1172.

Wadhera, A., Fazio, M., Bricca, G., & Stanton, O. (2006). Metastatic basal cell carincoma: A case report and literature review. How accurate is our incidence data? *Dermatology Online Journal*, Vol. 12, No. 5, (September 2006), pp. 7.

Warner, CL & Cockerell, CJ. (2011). The new 7th edition American Joint Committee On Cancer staging of cutaneous non-melanoma skin cancer: a critical review. *American Journal of Clinical Dermatology*, Vol. 12, No. 3, (June 2011), pp. 147-154.

Woods, RL. & Steward, JF. (1980). Metastatic basal cell carcinoma: report of a case responding to chemotherapy. *Postgraduate Medical Journal*, Vol. 56, No. 654, (May 1980),pp. 272-273.

6

Genomics of Basal and Squamous Cell Carcinomas

Venura Samarasinghe[1,2], John T. Lear[1,2], Vishal Madan[1,2]
[1]*The Dermatology Centre, Hope Hospital, Manchester*
[2]*Central Manchester Dermatology Centre, Manchester*
UK

1. Introdcution

Non-melanoma skin cancers, which include basal and squamous cell cancers, are the most common human cancers. Because of their relatively low metastatic rate and relatively slow growth these are frequently underreported. The high prevalence and the frequent occurrence of multiple primary tumours in affected individuals make non-melanoma skin cancers an important but underestimated public health problem.

There has been a dramatic increase in the incidence of non-melanoma skin cancer in the past 40 to 50 years, despite the awareness of the harmful effects of excessive sun exposure. A population-based study from Wales has shown that the crude incidence for non-melanoma skin cancer has increased from 173.5 to 265.4 per 100,000 population per annum between 1988 and 1998 (Holme *et al, 2000, Br J Dermatol).*

Although ultraviolet radiation is the most important risk factor in the genesis of both squamous cell carcinomas and basal cell carcinomas, there is a proportionately greater effect of increasing sun exposure on the risk of developing squamous cell carcinoma (Kricker *et al, 1995, Int J Cancer).* The desirability of a tan, increased leisure time and the introduction of cheap package holidays have resulted in a marked increase in the levels and change of pattern of sun exposure in the last 4 to 5 decades and this is thought to have led to an increase in the incidence of NMSC.

Basal cell carcinomas (BCC) which are the commonest cancer in Caucasians are slow growing tumour which, rarely metastasize. Their incidence is increasing by ~10%/year worldwide indicating that the prevalence of this tumour will soon equal that of all other cancers combined (*Karagas et al, 1995, Skin cancer: Mechanisms and human relevance*). Furthermore, 40-50% of patients will develop at least one more within 5 years.

UV radiation is the major aetiological agent in the pathogenesis of BCC and an understanding of its effects on the skin is clearly critical. However, though exposure to UVR is essential, its relationship with risk is unclear and epidemiological studies suggest its quantitative effect is modest. For example, a large European case-control study has shown only a two-fold increase in risk with increased exposure (*Rosso et al, 1996, Br J Can*) while recent studies suggest that intermittent rather than cumulative exposure is more important

(*Kricker, 1995, Int J Cancer*). The relationship between tumour site and exposure to UVR is also unclear. The distribution of lesions does not correlate well with the area of maximum exposure to UVR in that BCC are common on the eyelids, at the inner canthus and behind the ear, but uncommon on the back of the hand and forearm. Indeed, compared with squamous cell cancer (SCC), BCC are relatively more common on less exposed sites such as the trunk. Thus, though exposure to UVR is critical, patients develop BCC at sites generally believed to suffer relatively less exposure. The basis of the different susceptibility of skin at different sites to BCC development is not known, but may be related to the association of BCC with intermittent UV exposure.

Surgery remains the mainstay in the treatment of BCC. However, with a better understanding of the aetiopathogenesis and the relatively non- aggressive nature of these lesions, newer forms of destructive and non- destructive treatments are a focus of research. Induction of apoptosis, modulation of differentiation and immunomodualtion are some of the strategies by which some of the current pharmacotherapeutic agents exert their action. Unravelling the genetics of BCC will provide a basis for further research on the introduction of pharmacogenetics and development of newer agents targeting the specific genes implicated in the causation of BCC.

Chronic irritation, inflammation and injury to the skin can predispose to malignant epithelial neoplasms, in particular **squamous cell carcinomas** (*Kaplan, 1987, Adv Derm*). Examples include complicated scars from frostbite, electrical injury, chronic sinuses or fistulas, chronic osteomyelitis, chronic stasis dermatitis, and scars following various cutaneous infections.

The most often reported dermatoses complicated by cancer are discoid lupus erythematosus, scarring variants of epidermolysis bullosa, genital lichen sclerosus et atrophicus, its variant balanitis xerotica obliterans and lichen planus.

Lupus vulgaris, a chronic form of cutaneous tuberculosis is complicated by squamous cell carcinoma or less commonly basal cell carcinomas in up to 8% of the patients (Betti *et al 2002, Hautarzt, Forstrum et al, 1969, Ann Clin Res*). Squamous cell cancers can also arise from lesions of erythema *ab igne*, a characteristic dermatosis resulting from repeated or prolonged exposure to infrared radiation, insufficient to produce a burn (*Peterkin, 1955, BMJ*).

There is strong evidence that Photochemotherapy (PUVA) increases the risk of developing squamous cell carcinoma and this correlates with the cumulative dose of ultraviolet A. High dose PUVA (more than 200 treatments) is associated with a 14- fold increase in the risk of NMSC compared to low dose PUVA (*Stern et al, 1998 Arch Dermatol*). Arsenic is an important chemical carcinogen implicated in the development of non-melanoma skin cancer. In the first half of the 20th century, this was caused by the ingestion of medicinal arsenic in the form of medications for asthma and psoriasis. Mining and well water which is high in arsenic are the main sources today.

Patients who have received a renal transplant have a 50-250-fold increased risk of developing squamous cell carcinoma and a 5 -10 fold increase in the risk of developing basal cell carcinoma implicating anti-tumour immunity (McGregor *et al, 1995, Lancet,* Bouwes Bavinck , *1995, Hum Exp Toxicol*). Moreover, there is a close association between the development of non-melanoma skin cancer and premalignant lesions such as actinic keratoses and the presence of viral warts in these patients (Bouwes Bavinck , *1995, Hum Exp Toxicol*). Actinic keratoses are hyperkeratotic lesions occurring on chronic light exposed adult skin, and carry a low risk of progression to invasive squamous cell carcinoma. Lesions are usually multiple and comprise of macules or papules with a rough scaly surface resulting from disorganised keratinisation and a variable degree of inflammation. Although the rate of progression of individual squamous cell carcinoma has been estimated to be less than 0.1%, the presence of actinic keratoses is an important marker of excessive UV exposure and increased risk of non-melanoma skin cancer (Salasche, *2000, J Am Acad Dermatol)*

Mucosal lesions such as leukoplakias are also known to be premalignant with 2-5 % becoming malignant in 10 years (*Crispian, 2004, Rooks textbook of Dermatology, Blackwell publishing*). Bowen's disease is a form of intraepidermal squamous cell carcinoma, which presents as a persistent, non-elevated, red, scaly or crusted plaque and carries a small potential of invasive spread. Most studies suggest a risk of invasive cancer of about 3%. There is a significant frequency of multiple lesions and an association of Bowen's disease with other skin cancers, which may reflect predominant solar aetiology or, in some cases exposure to arsenic. Genital, especially perianal Bowen's disease has a higher risk of invasive malignancy.

Various studies indicate that the risk of skin cancer may be related to the overall amount of immunosupression (Jensen , *1999, Science,* Bouwes Bavinck ,*1996,* Transplantation, Dantal , *1998, Lancet*). Skin cancers are the most common malignancies that occur in transplant patients and their frequency increases with time after transplantation (Penn, *1993,*Hematol Oncol Clin North Am). The normal SCC/BCC ratio as observed in normal population is reversed in transplant recipients, with an excess in SCC development (Ong *et al, 1999, J Am Acad Dermatol,* Barr *et al, 1989, Lancet*) Moreover, these tumours behave more aggressively with a higher risk of metastasis than in general population (Penn , *1991,Transplant Proc*).

Patients receiving renal transplant from HLA -B antigen mismatched donors, are at a higher risk of developing SCC, which is thought to be related to more intense immunosupression which these patients receive (Bouwes Bavinck *et al 1991,*N Engl J Med.). SCC in transplant patients develop mostly on sun exposed sites (Bavinck *et al 1993,*Br J Dermatol.) and are more frequent in individuals with fair skin, blue eyes, and blonde and red hair (Bavinck *et al 1993,*Br J Dermatol., Euvrard *et al 1995, J Am Acad Dermatol,* McLelland *et al 1998,*Transplantation.); the standard risk factors for development of SCC. Early diagnosis and treatment of squamous cell cancers is important to avoid metastasis and tissue destruction as these cancers are more invasive and have a higher metastatic spread compared to basal cell cancers.

2. SCC predisposing syndromes

2.1 Xeroderma pigmentosum

An autosomal recessive disease characterised by elevated sensitivity to sunlight, multiple epidermal skin cancers in childhood as a consequence of increased susceptibility to DNA damage and abnormal DNA repair. In vitro, cells from XP patients show a decreased ability to conduct base excision repair in which single strand areas of DNA are excised and replaced with a new set of bases after sunlight induced damage.

2.2 Albinism

Partial or complete failure to produce melanin in the skin and the eyes. SCC and melanoma develop in sun exposed sites of most individuals at an early age. (Lookingbill *et al 1995,* J Am Acad Dermatol.)

2.3 Muir Torre syndrome

Germ line mutations in genes involved in DNA mismatch repair and microsatellite instability result in this autosomal dominant syndrome characterised by the presence of one or more sebaceous neoplasms in association with internal malignancy, most frequently of the colon. SCC have also been described in these patients.

2.4 KID (Keratosis, Icthyosis, Deafness)

Invasive SCC developing within dysplastic lesions have been reported in several patients suffering from this syndrome (Madariaga *et al, 1986,*Cancer).

2.5 Dystrophic epidermolysis bullosa

Recessive dystrophic epidermolysis bullosa (RDEB) is an autosomal recessive mechano-bullous disorder caused by mutations in the human type VII collagen gene (COL7A1). Individuals with DEB lack type VII collagen and anchoring fibrils, structures that attach epidermis and dermis. The leading cause of death in RDEB is invasion and metastasis of cutaneous SCC. Although the SCC in RDEB are frequently well-differentiated by histopathology, they often have a poor prognosis due to multicentricity, rapid invasiveness, and development of distant metastases. Mutations in the p53 tumor suppressor gene and loss of p16ink4a through hypermethylation have been seen in cutaneous SCC from these patients (Arbiser *et al, 2004,* J Invest Dermatol). This suggests that alterations in both p53 and p16ink4a can contribute to SCC in RDEB. Patients with RDEB have also been found to have elevated levels of b fibroblast growth factor, which may contribute to increased fibroblast collagenase and the development of SCC (Arbiser *et al, 1998,* Mol Med). Reduced expression of IGFBP-3, as seen in SCC associated with RDEB, has been suggested as a likely reason for the aggressive behaviour and poor prognosis of these tumors (Mallipeddi *et al, 2004,* J Invest Dermatol).

2.6 Fanconi anaemia

Fanconi anemia is an autosomal recessive disorder characterized by congenital malformations, bone marrow failure, and the development of SCC and other cancers. Environmental factor such as human papillomavirus (HPV) may be involved in the pathogenesis of SCC in Fanconi anemia patients (Kutler *et al 2003,* J Natl Cancer Inst). HPV DNA was isolated in 84% of the SCC specimens from the patients with Fanconi anaemia and a large proportion of patients with Fanconi anemia and SCC were homozygous for Arg72, a p53 polymorphism that may be associated with increased risk for HPV-associated human malignancies (Kutler *et al 2003,*J Natl Cancer Inst).

2.7 Rothmund Thompson syndrome

Rothmund-Thomson syndrome (RTS) is a rare autosomal recessive genodermatosis characterized by early onset of progressive poikiloderma including alopecia, dystrophic teeth and nails, juvenile cataracts, short stature, hypogonadism, bone defects and several other cutaneous and extracutaneous findings. Most (but apparently not all) cases of RTS are caused by null or hypomorphic mutations in the *RECQL4* gene, a putative DNA helicase. A role for RECQL4 in the repair of DNA double-strand breaks by homologous recombination has been suggested (Petkovic *et al, 2005 J Cell Sci*). Several cases of skin malignancies including SCC have been described in RTS patients, indicating a higher incidence of cutaneous malignancies (Piquero-Casals *et al 2002,*Pediatr Dermatol).

2.8 Werner syndrome

Werner syndrome is a genetic disorder of early ageing, excess cancer risk, high incidence of type II diabetes mellitus, early atherosclerosis, ocular cataracts, and osteoporosis. The protein encoded by the defective gene, WRN (WRNp) associates with 3'-5'-exonuclease and ATPase activities. Werner syndrome protein (WRN) is a RecQ-type DNA helicase, which seems to participate in DNA replication, double-strand break (DSB) repair, and telomere maintenance. A deficiency in maintaining DNA integrity is thought to be a consequence of the defective DNA helicase. In vivo alterations of oxidative stress parameters in WS patients have been demonstrated which may cause oxidative damage to biomolecules, with multiple oxidative stress-related alterations, resulting in multi-faceted clinical consequences (Pagano *et al, 2005,* Biogerontology, Pagano *et al, 2005,* Free Radic Res).

2.9 Other syndromes

These include hereditary non-polyposis coli, dyskeratosis congenita, Huriez syndrome and chronic mucocutaneous candidiasis.

3. Candidate susceptibility genes

The concept of genetic susceptibility to BCC and SCC is complex as genes may influence susceptibility as well as tumour numbers, rate of appearance and site. Selection of putative susceptibility genes must be in part subjective though the varied effects of UVR suggest that candidate genes may be selected from those involved in DNA repair, defence against oxidative stress, immune modulation, tanning and other related biochemical activities.

Although sunlight plays a crucial role in the development of SCC and to a lesser extent BCC, there is enough evidence that this is process is multifactorial with contributions from genetic and environmental factors. Several genes have been implicated in providing protection against and modifying the effects of UV radiation. It is also understood that UV is both mutagenic and locally immunosuppressant, thereby implying a huge pathogenic potential.

3.1 DNA repair

Signature UV-DNA lesions, cyclobutane dimers and 6-4 photoproducts, are repaired via the nucleotide excision repair pathway which may be subdivided into transcription-coupled repair and global genome repair. The XPC protein is specific to this latter repair pathway recognizing helix distorting lesions and initiating their repair. Inactivating XPC mutations are associated with xeroderma pigmentosa and an extremely high risk of skin cancer. Most early research on DNA repair and skin cancer was performed in patients with xeroderma pigmentosum (XP), a rare autosomal recessive syndrome in which multiple skin tumours are seen. Reduced capacity to repair DNA was observed in XP cells (*Cleaver et al, 1969, Proc Natl Acad Sci USA*). Early in life, homozygote XP patients develop severe photosensitivity and a 2,000-fold increased risk of skin cancer.

A common polymorphism in intron 9 of the XPC gene has been associated with both reduced repair of UV-DNA damage and increased risk of squamous cell head and neck cancer. It has been reported that PAT+ polymorphism may slightly modify the risk of SCC among individuals with a phenotype which results in low UV-DNA adduct burdens (Nelson *et al, 2005,* Cancer Let*t*). The XPD is another gene involved in the nucleotide excision repair pathway removing DNA photoproducts induced by UV radiation. Genetic variation in XPD may exert a subtle effect on DNA repair capacity with an inverse association between the Lys751Gln and Asp312Asn polymorphisms and the risks of melanoma and squamous cell carcinoma (*Han et al, 2005,* Cancer Epidemiol Biomarkers Prev).

UVA-induced oxidative DNA damage and blocked DNA replication by UVB-induced photoproducts can lead to double-strand breaks (DSBs). DSB repair genes XRCC2, XRCC3, and LigaseIV were evaluated for their associations with skin cancer risk. (*Han et al, 2004,*Cancer Res). XRCC3 18085T (241Met) allele and its associated haplotype were significantly inversely associated with the risks of SCC and BCC (*Han et al, 2004,* Br J Cancer) The XRCC1 gene is also involved in the base excision repair pathway. The 399Gln allele was inversely associated with SCC risk in those who had five or more lifetime sunburns, those with a family history of skin cancer, and those in the highest tertile of cumulative sun exposure in a bathing suit (*Han et al 2004,* Cancer Res.). There was also a significant association of the carriage of 194Trp allele with increased SCC risk, which was modified by family history of skin cancer (*Han et al, 2004,* Cancer Epidemiol Biomarkers Prev).

In sporadic BCC, DNA repair capacity below the upper 30th percentile was associated with a 2.3 fold increase in BCC relative risk. However, some studies have reported increased repair in BCC patients and so batch variability and the effects of age, family history of skin cancer and current sun exposure may confound results (*Hall et al 1994, Int J Cancer*). At least two types of XP are caused by defects in DNA helicases that are involved in nucleotide excision repair and in transcription. Werner and Bloom syndromes are hereditary skin cancer disorders that are associated with helicase defects but curiously not with the development of BCC's (*Yu Ce et al, 1996, Science, Ellis et al, 1995, Cell*). Rothmund-Thomsen syndrome, which in some cases is caused by defects in a DNA helicase (*Kitao et al, 1999, Nat Genet*) does seem to predispose to BCC (*Wang et al, 2001, Am J Med Genet*). This tissue specific effect of helicases is poorly understood. Also, other forms of genomic instability disorders including the chromosome breakage disorders like ataxia telangiectasia and Nijmegen breakage syndrome and disorders with p53 gene mutations like Li Fraumeni syndrome (*Malkin et al, 1990, Science*) or dyskeratosis congenita, a disorder associated with failure to maintain telomeres (*Knight et al, 1999, Am J Hum Genet, Vulliamy T, 2001, Nature*) are not causally associated with BCC.

3.2 Chemical detoxication

While exposure to UVR is accepted as a critical causative factor in the pathogenesis of BCC, the magnitude of the risk associated with increased exposure appears to be insufficiently large to explain the considerable phenotypic diversity demonstrated by patients in terms of tumour numbers, site and patterns of presentation.

UVA and UVB radiation cause indirect damage to DNA by inducing oxidative stress (*Griffiths et al, 1998,* Crit Rev Clin Lab Sc*i*). Reactive oxygen species thus produced, interact with lipids, proteins and DNA to generate intermediates that combine with DNA to form adducts (*Lear et al, 2000,* Br J Dermatol).

The authors have focused on the extensive clinical diversity following initial presentation, demonstrated by patients to identify subgroups that are associated with different risks of developing tumours. Two phenotypes are particularly important; firstly, presentation with clusters of BCC. These patients, termed multiple presentation phenotypes (MPP), had 2-5 BCC at one presentation and comprised 15% of our study group of 1200 BCC patients. A minority of patients demonstrated multiple clustering events, a phenomenon that appears to be strongly associated with a genetic pre-disposition (*Ramachandran et al, 1999, Cancer Epidemiol Biomarkers Prev; Ramachandran et al, 2000, Cancer*).

The second risk phenotype, characterized by tumours on the trunk, is also associated with a pre-disposition. These patients are important as there is evidence that different mechanisms mediate development of BCC on this, compared with other sites. For example, patients whose first tumour was truncal had more BCC than other patients (mean 2.4 vs. 2.0 tumours), were significantly younger at first presentation and developed more clusters of BCC than cases who did not develop truncal tumours. First presentation with a truncal tumour is associated with significantly more subsequent BCC on this site compared with cases with an initial head and neck lesion (*Ramachandran et al, 2001, Cancer*). These data suggest the development of a truncal BCC is not random but rather is associated with a pre-disposition. In contrast, the rate of increase of non-truncal BCC/year was similar in patients with and without initial truncal lesions suggesting different mechanisms determine the development of truncal and non-truncal BCC (*Ramachandran et al, 2001, Cancer*).

Both the MPP and truncal phenotypes were characterized by a susceptibility to develop numerous BCC. All patients with more than 5 BCC had one or both of these phenotypes.

The GST supergene family offers protection against cytotoxic and mutagenic effects of electrophiles generated by UV induced oxidative stress. This is achieved by conjugation of glutathione to electrophiles. GSTM1 catalyses the conjugation of 4-hydroxynonenal and linoleic acid hydroperoxide, products of lipid peroxidation (*Kerb et al, 1997, J Invest Dermatol*). It also catalyses the conjugation of DNA hydroperoxide (*Kerb et al, 1997,J Invest Dermatol*), a product of DNA oxidation, 5 hydroxymethyluracil , a mutagenic compound formed by either oxidative attack on the methyl group of the thymine base of DNA or from deamination of products formed by the oxidation of 5-methylcytosine (*Boorstein at al 1989,* Nucleic Acids Res. *Lear JT et al 2000,*Br J Dermatol). The GSTM1 and GSTT1 have been shown to be associated with the development and accrual of basal cell carcinoma (*Lear et al 1996, 1997, Carcinogenesis*), raising the possibility of an association with SCC as well. Indeed,

GSTM1 gene has been shown to be associated with actinic keratoses, supporting the possibility of its implication in SCC (Carless *et al, 2002,* J Invest Dermatol.).

The authors have examined the role of polymorphism in genes encoding detoxifying enzymes such as glutathione S-transferases (GST) and cytochrome P450s (CYP). The CYP supergene family comprise over 30 isoforms, which catalyse the biotransformation of a range of xenobiotics, often as the first of a two-phase detoxication. The resultant potentially highly reactive intermediate is then a substrate for phase two enzymes including members of the GST supergene family. The GSTs can also catalyse the detoxication of the products of oxidative stress (e.g. lipid and DNA hydroperoxides). Cytosolic GST activity in mammalian tissues is due to the presence of multiple GST isozymes, which can be assigned to 8 classes, e.g. α, θ, μ, π σ,κ,ω and ζ (*Hayes et al, 1995, Crit Rev Biochem Mol).* In human skin, the π class of GST is the predominant isozymes and is found predominantly in sebaceous glands (*Raza et al, 1991, J Invest Dermatol*). GST- π has been suggested to be an oncofetal protein that is expressed during carcinogenesis (*Moscow et al, 1998, Proct Natl Acad Sci USA*). Several polymorphisms in GST family members exist (*Hayes et al, 1995, Crit Rev Biochem Mol Biol; Pemble , 1994,Biochem J*) and have been associated with impaired detoxification, thus influencing the risk for several cancers, including non-melanoma skin cancer (*Heagerty et al, 1994, Lancet; Heagerty , 1996, Br J Cancer*).

A GSTT1 null genotype is associated with high UV sensitivity (*Kerb et al, 1997 J Invest Dermatol*) and we have shown that a GSTM1 null genotype also predisposes for BCC, probably due to its role in defence against UV induced oxidative stress (*Learet al, 1997, Carcinogenesis; Lear, 1996,Carcinogenesis*). Polymorphism of GSTM3 was also shown to increase the risk for multiple BCC (*Yengi, 1996, Cancer Res*). Polymorphism in cytochrome p450 CYP2D6 has also been associated with susceptibility as well as tumour numbers (together with vitamin D receptor and tumour necrosis factor alpha). In the case of multiple clustering, associations between the CYP2D6 EM genotype and risk demonstrated particularly large odds ratio (OR=15.5) (*Ramachandran et al, 1999, Cancer Epidemiol Biomarkers Prev; Lear et al, 1996, Carcinogenesis*).

3.3 Immunological effects

Though the role of UVR in the pathogenesis of skin tumours has been extensively studied, several reports have suggested that the resultant tumours are, at least in mice, highly immunogenic and regress on transfer to non-exposed hosts. This implies that the immune status of the UVR irradiated skin is compromised in those who develop tumours (*Granstein, 1996, Photochem Photobiol*). These findings are explained by data showing that exposure to UVR results in a cascade of events including a T-lymphocyte-mediated immunosuppression (*Kripke, 1994, Cancer Res; Streilein 1993, J Invest Dermatol*). The extent of the immunosuppression appears, to some degree, dose-dependent. Studies on the mechanism of this effect have concentrated on two chromophores; DNA and urocanic acid, both of which can result in altered expression of several cytokines including tumour necrosis factor alpha (TNF-α), interleukin (IL-)10, IL-1α/β, IL-3, IL-6, IL-8, IL-10, granulocyte-macrophage colony-stimulating factor (GM-CSF) and nerve growth factor. This results in an alteration from a T helper 1 (Th1) to a suppressive T helper 2 (Th2) response (*Granstein, 1996, Photochem Photobiol; Kripke, 1994, Cancer Res; Streilein 1993, J Invest Dermatol*) thereby inhibiting the ability of antigen presenting cells to induce anti-tumour immunity. In a pilot study, we found in 133 patients with multiple BCC, the TNF allele haplotype a2b4d5 significantly influenced BCC number (mean BCC number; 8.1 vs. 3.7 in other allele combinations) (*Hajeer et al, 2000, Br J Dermatol*). Further support for the role of the immune system in the pathogenesis of skin cancer came from the finding that HLA-DR4 is associated with multiple BCC (Czarnecki *et al, 1993, Dermatology*) but this has been disputed (*Rompel et al, 1995, Rec Res Canc Res*). Interestingly, there is a possible link between GST and immune modulation in non-melanoma skin cancer with studies showing a link between contact hypersensitivity to dinitrochlorobenzene (a substrate for GST) and squamous cell carcinoma (and non-significantly with BCC) (*de Berker , 1995, Lancet*). Furthermore, GSTM1 and GSTT1 genotypes have been shown to influence inflammatory response following UVR exposure, a finding possibly reflecting the link between oxidative stress and eicosanoid mobilisation.

3.4 Immunosuppression

The critical role of immunomodulation in skin cancer susceptibility is further supported by data showing immunosuppressed transplant patients are at considerably higher risk of both BCC and SCC than the general population. SCC of the skin is the most common malignancy occurring in the setting of solid organ transplantation and immunosuppression, and its incidence increases substantially with the extended survival after transplantation (*Otley et al, 2000, Liver Transpl*). SCC occurs more frequently in transplant patients (*Ondrus et al, 1999, Int Urol Nephrol*) whereas in the general populations BCC is three to six times more frequent than SCC (*Barrett et al, 1993, Cancer*). It was shown in heart transplant recipients that the number of skin cancers is significantly correlated with both age at transplantation and duration of follow -up (*Ong, 1999, J Am Acad Dermatol*). In Europe, 40% of renal transplant recipients develop skin cancer within 20 years after grafting, (*Hartevelt et al, 1990, Transplantation*). Heart transplant recipients are at a higher risk than kidney transplant recipients, most probably due to the fact that they receive higher doses of immunosuppression agents (*Euvrard et al, 1995, J Am Acad Dermatol*) but it cannot be overlooked that the different types of immunosuppressive agents have different effects in this respect. Immunosupression as practised after organ transplantation does not increase the risk of developing BCC to the same extent as SCC. The incidence of BCC seems not to be affected by PUVA treatment. A diminished response to skin application of dinitrochlorobenzene was found in people with SCC but not in patients with BCC, again supporting the notion that the incidence of BCC is not affected by immune status to the same extent as SCC (*de Berker et al, 1995, Lancet*).

3.5 Human Immunodeficiency Virus

People suffering from aquired immunodeficiency syndrome (AIDS) have shown an elevated risk for the development of BCC (*Franceschi et al, 1998, Br J Cancer; Ragni et al, 1993, Blood*). Human Immunodeficieny virus (HIV) patients with BCC more frequently show blue eyes, blonde hair, family history and extensive prior sun-exposure (*Lobo et al, 1992, Arch Dermatol*). The pigmentation phenotype is probably an independent risk factor that adds to the increased risk of BCC conferred by the immunosuppression. There have been some reports of BCC's metastasising in people suffering from AIDS, (*Steigleder, 1987, Z Hautkr; Sitz, 1987, JAMA*) suggesting that immune surveillance is one of the factors determining the normally metastatic nature of the BCC. Why immunosuppression by HIV increases the risk of BCC, where as pharmaceutical immunosuppression does not is not clear. The depletion of CD4 lymphocytes by HIV may lead to a more pervasive defect in adaptive antitumour immunity that does mere functional suppression by commonly used immunosuppressive compounds.

3.6 Human Leukocyte Antigen (HLA) haplotypes

The major histocompatibility complex (MHC) genes code for membrane protein that play important roles in controlling immune responses (*Benacerraf, 1981, Science*). There are two classes of genes, class I (HLA-A, -B, -C) and class II (HLA-DR, -DP and DQ) which play a role in host defence against the development and spread of tumours (*Dausset et al, 1982, Cancer Surv*). For example, loss of class 1 antigens is related to tumour progression in melanomas (*Ruiter, 1984, Cancer Res*). Furthermore, abnormalities in cell- mediated immunity have been reported in patients with multiple BCC (*Myskowsky et al, 1981, J Am Acad Dermatol*) whereas normal skin shows high levels of class 1 molecules, BCC shows either complete absence or heterogeneous expression (*Cabrera et al, 1992, Immunobiol*). All class I –negative tumours were histologically proven to be aggressive, whereas all non-aggressive BCC's were class I positive. The low levels or absence of expression of class I antigens may result in escape from recognition by cytotoxic T cells, which then facilitates tumour growth. (*Garcia- Plata, 1991, Inv Met*). The presence of HLA – DR7 and decrease of HLA-DR4 are significantly associated with BCC (*Bouwes Bavinck, 2000, Arch Dermatol*). HLA -DR4 is decreased in BCC, especially in patients with multiple BCC's located on the trunk (*Rompel et al, 1995, Rec Res Canc Res,*). HLA-DR1 is weakly associated with the development of multiple BCC's at an early age (*Czarnecki et al, 1992, J Am Acad Dermatol*). A correlation between HLA-A11 expression and skin cancer in immunosuppressed renal transplant recipients has been shown (*Bavnick, 1990, N Engl J Med; Bouwes Bavnick, 1997, Australia J Invest Dermatol*). One study showed that HLA –A11 was associated with resistance to skin cancer in renal transplant recipients, (*Bavnick, 1990, N Engl J Med*) while another study shows that renal transplant recipients with HLA – A11 had an increased risk for developing skin cancer (*Bouwes Bavnick, 1997, Australia J Invest Dermatol*). The apparent discrepancy may be the result of different genetic backgrounds and differential environmental factors.

3.7 Human Papilloma Virus

The life cycle of these species-specific DNA tumour viruses is inseparably linked to differentiation processes in pluristratified epithelia (Stanley *et al, 1994,* Ciba Found Symp). Mucosal HPV types 16, 18, 31 and 33 are strongly associated with the genesis of anogenital and cervical carcinomas (*Bosch et al, 2002,* J Clin Pathol). Following viral genome integration, E6 and E7 oncoproteins are overexpressed, with inhibition of apoptosis via p53 dependent and independent mechanisms (*Thomas et al, 1999,* Oncogene). E6 protein from the cervical associated HPC-16 mediates degradation of p53 (*Black et al, 2003,*Clin Exp Immunol). A common p53 polymorphism at position 72 replacing proline with arginine renders p53 more susceptible to E6 mediated degradation. The arginine allele was found to be a risk factor in the development of cervical cancers and there was also a significant association with cutaneous SCC development in renal transplant patients (*Storey et al, 1998,* Nature).

Cutaneous HPV types 5 and 8 are associated with warty lesions and SCC in the sun exposed sites of patients with the rare inherited condition epidermodysplasia verruciformis. This led to the proposal that these EV types may also be oncogenic. (*Majewski et al, 1995,* Arch Dermatol). The mechanism by which EV associated HPV might contribute to the development of SCC remains unclear. Unlike oncogenic mucosal HPV, EV-HPV DNA persist extrachromosomally in cancers and EV associated E6 proteins are unable to abrogate apoptosis via the degradation of p53. (*Elbel et al, 1997,*Virology) Instead, BAK protein, a member of the Bcl- 2 family may be abrogated resulting in inhibition of apoptosis (*Jackson et al 2000,* Genes Dev).

HPV DNA has been identified in over 80% of immunosuppressed and 30% of immunocompetent SCC patients and EV-HPV types are consistently overexpressed in immunosuppressed patients. (*Harwood et al, 2002,* Curr Opin Infect Dis, *Pfister et al 2003,* J Natl Cancer Inst Monogr.) The association between prevalence of EV-HPV infection and SCC risk has been further strengthened by seroepidemiological studies (*Bouwes Bavinck et al 2000,* Br J Dermatol., *Feltkamp et al, 2003,* Cancer Res. *Masini et al 2003,*Arch Dermatol.). Furthermore, localisation of HPV DNA to malignant keratinocytes in SCC as well as EV-HPV gene transcription in almost 40% of tumours has been found by in situ hybridisation technique, thus providing further evidence of the role of HPV in pathogenesis of SCC (*Purdie et al 2005,* J Invest Dermatol.). The presence of UV induced p53 mutations in cutaneous SCC contrasts with tumours induced by high-risk HPV types, which contain wild type p53. It is postulated that arginine allele of p53, perhaps in combination with UV induced mutation, is more susceptible to interference from particular HPV types and subsequent malignant transformation (*Black et al, 2003,*Clin Exp Immunol). HPV 77 has so far been detected in cutaneous lesions of renal transplant patients and contains a p53 DNA binding site. Besides inducing p53 mutations, sunlight may also be indirectly involved in the pathogenesis of SCC by causing activation of p53 and subsequent stimulation of HPV 77 promoter activity (*Purdie et al, 1999,* EMBO J.). Other viruses suggested to increase susceptibility to SCC include HPV 20, HPV 27 (Ruhland *et al 2001,*Int J Cancer.) and human herpes virus type 1 (*Leite et al 2005,* Cancer Lett.).Although HPV has been associated strongly with malignant progression of warts to SCC and with epidermodysplasia verruciformis, (*Galloway et al, 1989, Adv Virus Res*) different oncogenic subtypes of the virus were found in 60% of BCC's from immunosuppressed patients in contrast to 36% of BCC's from non-immunosuppressed patients, suggesting that these viruses may be involved in the development of BCC (*Shamanin et al, 1996, J Natl Cancer Inst*). In renal transplant recipients with skin cancer, HPV 5 /8 DNA could be detected, (*Barr et al, 1989, Lancet*) and Weinstock et al (*Weinstock et al, 1995, Arch Dermatol*) suggested immunosuppression to be a factor in BCC carcinogenesis by affecting HPV infection.

3.8 Delayed hypersensitivity

Patients with large SCC were found to have defective systemic cell-mediated immunity as shown by reduced reaction to intradermal antigen, and low rate of sensitization to dinitrochlorobenzene (DNCB) (Weimar *et al 1980,* J Am Acad Dermatol.). Because GST metabolises DNCB and polymorphisms of GST are associated with multiple skin tumours, variations in GST may underlie these differences (de Berker *et al, 1995, Lancet*). The T cell levels and leukocyte migration test in preoperative patients with SCC were also found to be significantly lower than in the noncancer control population. (Avgerinou *et al, 1985,* Dermatologica.)

4. Germline and somatic mutations

Carcinogenesis involves a stepwise progression from a normal to a malignant phenotype through an accumulation of genetic alterations to cellular proto-oncogenes, that stimulate cell proliferation and tumour suppressor genes (TSG) that inhibit this process. In tumours, mutation of proto-oncogenes results in expression of constitutively active proteins, whereas mutational inactivation of TSG leads to loss of protein function.

4.1 p53

p53 is a TSE that normally functions in cell-cycle arrest, DNA repair and apoptosis. It functions as a critical regulator of the cell cycle progression and programmed cell death in response to insults that damage DNA, such as UVR exposure (*Natraj, 1995,* Photochem Photobiol.). The p-53 gene encodes a phosphoprotein that is involved in cell-cycle control and maintenance of chromosomal stability (*Katayama 2004, Nat Genet; Hollstein M, 1991, Science*). The most common genetic aberrations in human skin cancers are found at the level of p53 gene expression (*Kastan, 1991, Cancer Res*). DNA strand breaks results in expression of p-53, which in turn stimulates p21 ^{Cip1} expression, which binds and inhibits cyclin-dependent kinases 2 and 4 resulting in G1 blockade of cell cycle progression. This inhibition of cell cycle progression allows for DNA repair before it is replicated in S phase to prevent retention of introduced mutations. In severe DNA damage, p53 induces BAX, which binds to BCL-2 and inhibits its antiapoptotic activity, resulting in programmed cell death. Thus, mutations would be retained in genomic DNA if p53 gene becomes inactivated, leading to clonal expansion and tumourigenesis.

p53 gets activated in response to cellular stress through phosphorylation (*Siliciano et al, 1997, Genes Dev, Caspari, 2000, Curr Biol*). MDM2 associates with p53 and regulated its level of activity depending on the phosphorylation status of p53. Upon dephosphorylation, p53 binds to MDM2 and is degraded through the ubiquitin-proteasome pathway (*Kubbutat et al, 1997, Nature, Haupt et al, 1997, Nature)*

The response to DNA damage is growth, senescence or apoptosis (*Vogt Sionov et al, 1999, Oncogene).* The relative cellular content of p53 determines the response following DNA damage; when the content is low to moderate, cells will go into cell- cycle arrest to allow DNA repair, but when p53 levels are high, cells will progress to apoptosis (*Ronen et al, 1996, Cell Growth Different*). In response to DNA damage, p53 is phosphorylated by DNA damage-sensing proteins such as ATM and becomes detached from MDM2, resulting in stabilization and activation and of target genes regulated by p53 (*Unger et al, 1999, EMBO J*). In normal skin, wild type p53 is not detectable but appears within 2 hours after UV irradiation, with peak levels at 24 hours and again undetectable levels at 36 hours (*Hall et al, 1993, Oncogene*). Mutant p53 can accumulate in cells and p53 mutations have been detected in about half of all BCCs (*Aeupemkiate et al, 2002, Histopathology, Demirkan et al, 2000, Pathol Oncol Res*). Aggressive BCC are significantly associated with increased p53 expression, probably representing the mutated form. Despite the available evidence, the apparent limited contribution of DNA damage and chromosomal instability to the BCC phenotype means that the relevance of p53 mutations for BCC growth remains to be demonstrated as in the absence of genetic damage p53 activation does not occur. Moreover, one of the hallmarks of p53 dysfunction, aberrant mitosis, has never been observed in BCC (*Pritchard, 1993, Am J Dermatopathol*).

Patients with BCC, who were sunscreen users, had significantly lower level of p53 mutations in their BCC as compared to non-sunscreen users (*Rosenstein el al, 1999,Photochem Photobiol*) suggesting that p53 mutations in BCC are secondary events. Inactivation of p53 occurs predominantly by point mutation of one of the allele followed by loss of the remaining wild type allele (*Knudson et al, 1985, Cancer Res*). The p53 gene shows UV signature mutation, i.e. predominantly C(C) → T (T) conversions (*Ziegler et al, 1993, Proct Natl Acad Sci USA, Wikonkal et al, 1999, J Invest Dermatol Symp Proc*). In 33% of BCCs found in Korean patients, p53 mutations were detected (*Kim, 2002, J Dermatol Sci*) and up to 50% of the BCCs in Caucasian patients showed this mutation (*Aeupemkiate et al, 2002, Histopathology, Demirkan, 2000, Pathol Oncol Res*), suggesting that different ethnic factors play a role in BCC carcinogenesis, although differences in sun exposure may account for some of the observed differences.

Thus, while it is known that *p53* is involved in genome surveillance through the regulation of cell proliferation and death and is frequently inactivated in BCC (*Rady et al, 1992 Cancer Res, Ziegler et al, 1993, Proct Natl Acad Sci USA*), with up to 56% of tumours displaying mutation in the conserved region of one *p53* allele, it has been suggested that *p53* mutation is a crucial but late event in BCC progression (*Van der Riet et al, 1994, Cancer Res*). BCC also display a high level of LOH specifically at chromosome 9q22 suggesting the existence of a BCC TSG in this region (*Quinn et al, 1994, Cancer Res*).

Up to 90% of cutaneous SCC lesions have UV induced signature mutations such as formation of thymidine dimers in the p53 gene, resulting in uncontrolled proliferation of keratinocytes (Brash et al, 1991, Proc Natl Acad Sci U S A, Ziegler, *1994,* Nature). Overexpression of p53 co-relates with sun-exposure (Coulter *et al 1995,* Hum Pathol. Liang , *1999,* Virchows Arch.) and mutant p53 has been observed to accumulate in the cell cytoplasm, probably due to increased half-life of the protein (Dowell *et al 1994,* Cancer Res, Soussi , *2000,* Ann N Y Acad Sci.). Indeed, sunlight- induced mutations are found in p53 in actinic keratoses, the precancerous lesion of for SCC. In addition, it has been shown that mutations at particular p53 codons are present in sun exposed normal human skin and UV irradiated mouse skin (Ziegler *et al, 1994,* Nature. Nakazawa *et al, 1994, Natl Acad Sci U SA,* Jonason *et al, 1996,* Proc Natl Acad Sci U S A.)

Sunlight has been shown to be a tumorigenic mutagen and tumour promoter by favouring the clonal expansion of p53 mutated cells. The role of UV in carcinogenesis is also supported by the observation that most human precancers (Marks *et al, 1986,* Br J Dermatol.) and UV induced clusters of p53 overexpressing cells in mouse skin (Berg *et al 1996,* Proc Natl Acad Sci U S A) regress in the absence of continued exposure. The dermal-epidermal junction and hair follicles are the locations of the presumed stem cells in skin (Lavker *et al 1993,* Recent Results Cancer Res.) and appear to be the source of tumours in experimental animals (Miller *et al,1993,* J Invest Dermatol.). It is therefore thought that normal sun exposed skin carries a substantial burden of keratinocyes predisposed to cancer (Jonason *et al, 1996,* Proc Natl Acad Sci U S A.). The ubiquitin proteasome pathway rapidly degrades wild type p53 in normal tissue (Maki *et al 1996,* Cancer Res.). Thus, high level of p53 expression is seen in cutaneous SCC and other tumours in contrast to the low levels found in non-malignant tissue.

Clonal expansion of p53 mutated cell would be favoured if a p53 mutation confers resistance to apoptosis resulting from UV exposure (Ziegler A, *1994,*Nature). Such resistance would allow sunlight to act as tumour promoter by killing normal cells and sparing the mutants (Ziegler A, *1994,*Nature.*)*. After surviving irradiation, these mutant cells could then clonally expand into vacated compartments (Jonason *et al, 1996,*Proc Natl Acad Sci U S A.).

4.2 p63

p63 is a p53 homologue that is mapped to chromosome 3q27. This gene encodes six different isoforms, which have either transactivating or dominant negative effects on p53-reporter genes. p63 is a reliable keratinocyte stem cell marker involved in the maintenance of the stem cell population . It is expressed in the nuclei of epidermal basal and suprabasal cells, cells of the germinative hair matrix and the external root sheath of hair follicles, basal cells of the sebaceous gland and in the myoepithelial /basal cells of the sweat glands. p63 has a nucleoplasmic distribution in the basal compartment of stratified epithelia such as skin, tonsil, bladder, and certain subpopulations of basal cells in prostate, breast, uterine cervix and bronchi (*Wang et al, 2001, Hum Pathol; Quade et al, 2001, Gynaecol Onco; Di Como et al, 2002, Clin Cancer Res*). All terminally differentiated cells stain negative for p63. The p63 is restricted to cells with high proliferation and absent from cells undergoing terminal differentiation (*Parsa et al, 1999, J Invest Dermatol*). p63-deficient mice have striking developmental defects such as absence or truncation of limbs, absence of hair follicles, teeth and mammary glands, and the skin lacks stratification and differentiation (*Mills et al, 1999, Nature*). This indicates that p63 is essential for several aspects of differentiation during embryogenesis. Several isoforms of p63 can bind to p53 consensus sequences and activate p53 target genes. p63 is only rarely mutated in BCC (*Little et al. , 2002, Int J Biochem Cell Biol*). p63 functions not only as a stem cell marker of keratinocytes but also maintain the stem cell phenotype. In keeping with its basal localisation in normal epidermis, BCC cells express p63 (*Di Como et al, 2002, Clin Cancer Res, Dellavale et al, 2002, Exp Dermatol*). It was shown that aberrant expression of p63 altered the UVB induced apoptotic pathway that down regulation of this protein in the response to UV irradiation is important in epidermal apoptosis (*Liefer et al, 2000, Cancer Res*).

Although it has been described that in contrast to p53, p63 seems not to be associated with tumor predisposition, as neither p63 knockout mouse models nor germline p63 mutations are related to an increased risk of tumourigenesis; its role in the pathogenesis of SCC is becoming more convincing. Using immunohistochemistry techniques undifferentiated cells of grade III SCCs showed strong positivity for p63 (Reis-Filho *et al 2002,* J Cutan Pathol.). The SCCs in situ showed remarkable expression of p63 in all cell layers. Terminally differentiated squamous cells were either negative or showed only focal immunoreactivity in the carcinomas. p63 is consistently expressed in the basal cells of epidermis and cutaneous appendages, including the basal/myoepithelial cells of sweat glands. These probabilities favour that p63 might play a role in the pattern of differentiation and in the oncogenesis of usual carcinomas of the skin (Reis-Filho *et al 2002,* J Cutan Pathol.).

4.3 PTCH

A major breakthrough in understanding BCC tumourigenesis came from the study of patients with Nevoid Basal Cell Carcinoma Syndrome (NBCCS) an autosomal dominant disease whose symptoms include developmental abnormalities and a predisposition to multiple BCC. The disease is linked to chromosome 9q22, which harbours the *PTCH* gene where inactivating germline mutations have been found in these patients (*Hahn et al, 1996, Cell; Johnson et al, 1996, Science*). Somatic *PTCH* mutation has also been described in sporadic BCC (*Azsterbaum et al, 1998, J Invest Dermatol, Gailani et al. 1996, Nat Genet*). In accordance with a tumour suppressor mechanism for *PTCH,* loss of the wild type allele has been demonstrated in BCC from both NBCCS patients and in up to 68% of sporadic BCC (*Gailani et al. 1996, Nat Genet*).

Although most SCC carry a mutation in the p53 gene, they have also been shown to display PTCH mutations (Ping *et al, 2001,*J Invest Dermatol.) and allelic loss of PTCH gene (Ahmadian *et al 1998,*Oncogene.) and an increased incidence of SCC has been observed in UV irradiated heterogeneous PTCH knock out mice (Aszterbaum *et al, 1999, Nat Med*). The introduction of wild-type PTCH into human SCC lines that express mutant PTCH has been shown to suppress their oncogenic potential (Koike *et al 2002,* Oncogene). These finding implicate the role of PTCH in development of SCC in addition to its established association with the development of BCC (Asplund *et al 2005,* Br J Dermatol.*)* However, the association between PTCH and cutaneous SCC development remains controversial as a previous investigation of the PTCH status in cutaneous SCC failed to identify mutations on such cases (Eklund *et al 1998*, Mol Carcinog). Consistently, PTCH LOH has not been found to be as frequent in SCC, indicating a lesser importance of PTCH gene in SCC development (Asplund *et al 2005,* Br J Dermatol.)

4.4 Hedegehog signalling and BCC development

PTCH is the human homologue of the *Drosophila patched* (*ptc)* gene which encodes Ptc protein. Ptc a part of a receptor for the diffusible morphagen Hedgehog (Hh). In *Drospophila* Hh signalling is essential for the control of segment polarity during development. Hh is expressed in the Hensen node, the floorplate of the neural tube, the early gut endoderm, the posterior limb buds and throughout the notochord, and encodes a signal responsible for patterning the early embryo (*Kim et al, 2002, J Dermatol Sci, Bodak et al, 1999, Proc Natl Acad Sci USA, Bale et al, 2001, Hum Mol Genet*).

Ptc negatively regulates Hh signalling through inhibition of a transmembrane signalling protein Smoothened (Smo). There is some evidence that Ptc may influence the localisation or intramembrane conformation of Smo (*Sprong et al, 2001, Nat Rev Mol Cell Biol*). Binding of Hh to Ptc releases Smo inhibition leading to intracellular signalling involving Costal-2, Fused and Suppressor of Fused proteins (*Stone et al, 1999, J Cell Sci*). This leads to activation of GSK3β which stimulated the release of a transcription factor Cubitus interrruptus (Ci) that regulates the expression of important genes involved in *Drosophila* cell proliferation including *dpp, wingless* and *ptc*. The Hh signalling pathway is highly conserved, where it is involved in determining cell fate and organogenesis in different species including humans (*Wicking et al, 1999, Oncogene*).

In humans, it is thought that signalling operates in a similar fashion to that described in *Drosophila*. To date, disrupted expression of the human homologues of *Hh* (*sonic hedgehog; SHH*), *Ptc (PTCH and PTCH2)*, *Smo* (*SMOH*) and *Ci (GLI)* have been demonstrated in BCC tumourigenesis. Overexpression of *SHH* in transgenic human skin induces features of BCC in mice (*Fan, 1997, Nat Med, Oro et al, 1997, Science*). Furthermore, *SHH* activating mutations have also been described in sporadic BCC (*Oreo et al, 1997, Science*). *SMOH* and *GLI* transgenic activation in mice leads to BCC-like cutaneous growths (*Xie et al, 1998, Nature, Nilsson et al 2000 Proc Natl Acad Sci. USA*). *SMOH, GLI-1* and *GLI-2* are frequently over expressed in BCC and *SMOH* activating mutations have also been described in 20% of sporadic BCC's (*Xie et al 1998, Nature; Kallassy, 1997 Cancer Res; Dahmane 1997, Nature; Grachtchou, ,2000, Nature Genet*). The consequences of deregulated Hh signalling are widespread, as the downstream targets of GLI transcription factors include *WNT* signalling (human homologue of *wingless*), *TGFß* (homologue of *dpp*) *BMP2B* and *BCL-2* (*Fan, 1997, Nature Med*) and may also influence cell cycle control genes including $p21^{WAF1}$ the *D-type cyclins* and *cyclin E* (*Fan, 1999, J Cell Biol; Duman-Scheel , 2002, Nature*).

4.5 Melanocortin-1 receptor genotype

As pigmentation influences NMSC risk, the identification of gene variants at the melanocortin-1 receptor (MC1R), which control the production of red pigmentation in Caucasian individuals, suggest that the allelic variation within this gene should likewise be associated with skin cancer risk (*Box et al 2001,*J Invest Dermatol.) Indeed, gene variations at this locus are important in determining susceptibility to melanoma, BCC, SCC and solar keratoses (*Box et al 2001,* J Invest Dermatol.). The association between MC1R variants and the propensity to develop solar lesions is mediated largely through three variants, Arg151Cys, Arg160Trp, and Arg294His, which are also associated with red hair, fair skin colour and tanning ability (Box *et al 2001,*J Invest Dermatol.).

4.6 RAS mutations

Although the role of TSG in the development of SCC is well established, evidence relating to the role of dominantly transforming oncogenes in the development of skin cancers is slow to emerge. Activating RAS mutations are the most common genetic abnormalities in human cancers. Following RAS mutation, MAPK mediated signalling and other pathways are activated, resulting in cell proliferation (Shields, *2000,* Trends Cell Biol.). Activation of RAS oncogenes usually occurs by point mutations within specific codons of the H-RAS, N-RAS, and K-RAS genes. Activating H-RAS mutations were observed in 35% to 46% of SCC (Kreimer-Erlacher, *2001,* Photochem Photobiol., Pierceall, *1991,*Mol Carcinog.) and 12% of actinic keratoses (Spencer *et al* , *1995,*Arch Dermatol.). Incidences and numbers of skin tumors were much greater in Hras128 rats (a transgenic rat line carrying 3 copies of the human c-Ha-ras proto-oncogene with its own promoter region) than in their wild-type counterparts (Park *el al, 2004,* Cancer Sci.)

These data suggest that RAS mutations play an important role in the pathogenesis of SCC.

4.7 CDKN2A

The p16(INK4a) and p14(ARF) TSGs are encoded within the CDKN2A locus on chromosome 9p21 and function as cell cycle regulatory proteins in the p53 and RB pathways. Loss of heterozygosity of 9p21 markers has been seen in some cases of SCC (Brown *et al 2004*). Mutational analysis has confirmed point mutations that changed the amino acid sequence of p16 (INK4a) and p14 (ARF). Promoter methylation of p16 (INK4a) and p14 (ARF) has also been detected. Absent protein expression was has been confirmed by immunohistochemistry in SCC with biallelic inactivating events. Overall, promoter methylation is the commonest mechanism of gene inactivation. Alterations at this locus are significantly more common in tumors from immunocompetent compared with immunosuppressed individuals (Brown *et al 2004,* J Invest Dermatol.). UV radiation-induced mutations in INK4a-ARF have been demonstrated in XP-associated skin carcinomas. The simultaneous inactivation of p53 and INK4a-ARF may be linked to the genetic instability caused by XP and could be advantageous for tumour progression.

4.8 Progression and initiation of BCC

Exposure to UVR is significant in BCC formation and this is reflected in the *p53* mutations identified; C-T and CC-TT transitions at di-pyrimidine sites. A third of the BCC displaying LOH at 9q reveal mutations to *PTCH* indicative of UVR exposure. However, most mutations to *PTCH* are not typical of exposure. Further, inactivation of the second *PTCH* allele through LOH is unlikely to be due to UVB (*Gailani et al, 1996, J Natl Cancer Inst*). In addition, *ptc* heterozygous knockout mice (*ptc/ptc*-) display features of NBCCs syndrome, these mice develop microscopic follicular neoplasms similar to trichoblastoma and 40% subsequently develop BCC. If exposed to ionising or UVR irradiation these neoplasms occur at a much earlier stage and there is a clear shift in histological features to BCC (*Aszterbaum et al, 1999, Nature Med*). Thus, whilst UVR exposure is critical to SCC development, it appears that in BCC, UVR exposure may be more important in modifying tumour progression. Further characterisation of the role of the Hh signalling pathway should provide new insights into BCC carcinogenesis. Identifying the mutations to these BCC genes and the relationship of these mutations to environmental carcinogens may explain the variation in phenotype of sporadic BCC. It is possible that mutations manifest different phenotypic effects depending on the genetic background of the patient (e.g. skin type, hair colour, GST genotype). Whilst gene mutation influences tumour development, we can speculate that inter-individual variation in genes that protect against exposure to environmental carcinogens may modify the effects of exposure to mutation in these target genes. Thus, we have found an increase in the incidence of tumour specific *p53* mutation and expression in ovarian cancer patients with *GSTM1* null genotype (*Sarhanis et al 1996, Br J Cancer*). In addition, CYP3A and CYP2D6 activities and the *GSTM1* null genotype have been associated with mutations to *p53* and *RB* and are associated with aggressiveness in bladder carcinoma (*Romkes et al, 1996, Carcinogenesis*).

5. Pharmacogenomics

As discussed above, UV radiation induced oxidative stress and mutagenic DNA lesions formed by reactive oxygen species (ROS) are pivotal in the pathogenesis of SCC. Clinical treatments inducing chronic oxidative stress may therefore carry a risk of therapy-related cancer. Immunosuppression by azathioprine (Aza) has been proposed as one such treatment. Biologically relevant doses of ultraviolet A (UVA) generate ROS in cultured cells with 6-thioguanine substituted DNA and 6-thioguanine and UVA are synergistically mutagenic (O'Donovan *et al, 2005,* Science.).

Kidney transplant recipients receiving cyclosporine, azathioprine, and prednisolone have a significantly (2.8 times) higher risk of cutaneous SCC relative to those receiving azathioprine and prednisolone alone (Jensen *et al, 1999, Am Acad Dermatol*) suggesting a tumourigenic role of cyclosporine based immunosuppressive therapy. Both cyclosporine and ascomycin inhibit removal of cyclobutane pyrimidine dimers, and UVB-induced apoptosis (Yarosh *et al, 2005,* J Invest Dermatol.). UVB induces nuclear localization of the transcription factor nuclear factor of activated T-cells (NFAT), a process blocked by cyclosporine and ascomycin (Yarosh *et al, 2005,* J Invest Dermatol.) These data suggest that the increased risk of skin cancer observed in organ-transplant patients may be as a result of not only systemic immune suppression but also the local inhibition of DNA repair and apoptosis in skin by calcineurin inhibitors(Yarosh DB *et al, 2005,* J Invest Dermatol.)

Thus, cancer is an increasingly recognized problem associated with immunosuppression. However, in contrast to cyclosporine which protects allografts from rejection but promotes cancer progression in transplant recipients, immunosuppressive agent rapamycin has been found to simultaneously protect allografts from rejection and attacks tumors in a complex transplant-tumor situation (Koehl *et al, 2004,*Transplantation.). In vitro experiments have shown that cyclosporine promotes angiogenesis by a transforming growth factor-beta-related mechanism, and that this effect is abrogated by rapamycin (Koehl *et al, 2004,* Transplantation.). Various surgical and non- surgical therapies are available for the treatment of BCC *(Albright et al, 1982, J Am Acad Dermatol*). In spite of the fact that surgical excision is still the most prominent therapy used, non –invasive therapies such as photodynamic therapy (PDT) (*Thissen et al, 2000, Br J Dermatol*), or topical application of 5-fluorouracil (5-FU) (Miller, *1997, J Am Acad Dermatol*) are currently becoming more and more interesting in selective cases, especially because of the improved cosmetic outcome.

5.1 Induction of apoptosis

Many currently used antineoplastic agents exert their therapeutic effects through the induction of apoptosis. Different cell types vary profoundly in their susceptibility, suggesting the existence of distinct cellular thresholds for apoptosis induction (*Fisher, 1994, Cell*). For example, BCC cells overexpressing IL-6 are resistant to UV irradiation and PDT –induced apoptosis (*Jee et al, 2001, Oncogene*). de novo p53 synthesis or stabilisation of p-53 is essential to induce apoptosis in BCC (*Jee et al, 1998, J Invest Dermatol*). Overexpression of the antiapoptotic bcl-2 has also been linked to resistance of cancers to various chemotherapeutic drugs (*Huang, 2000, Oncogene*). In BCC, interferon (IFN)-α induces apoptosis and is thus effective in the treatment (*Rodriguez- Villanueva et al, 1995, Int J Cancer*). Untreated BCC cells express FasL but not the receptor, but in IFN-α - treated BCC patients, the tumour cells express both FasL and receptor, whereas the peritumoural infiltrate mainly consists of Fas-receptor- positive cells (*Buechner, et al, 1997, J Clin Invest*). Therefore, with IFN- α treatment, BCC most likely regress through apoptosis.

The regression of tumours treated with 5-FU is probably caused by enhancing apoptosis in the tumour cells (*Brash, 1998, Cancer Surveys*). Apoptosis is involved in the regression of actinic keratoses after PDT (*Nakaseko et al, 2003, Br J Dermatol*).This therapy is also used for treatment of BCC, (*Kalka, 2000, J Am Acad Dermatol*), where tumour cells may also undergo apoptosis.

Phytochemicals known to induce apoptosis are also being applied in cancer prevention and therapy (*Hoffman et al, 1999, Cancer and the search for selective biochemical inhibitors, CRC Press*). In mice bearing skin tumours, tumour growth was inhibited by 70% after treatment with black tea, which was established by inhibition of proliferation and enhanced apoptosis (*Lu et al, 1997, Carcinogenesis*). Ajone, an organosulphur compound of garlic (*Apitz- Castro et al, 1988, Arznei-Mittelforschung*) has been shown to induce apoptosis in human promyeloleukaemic cells (*Dirsch, 1998, Mol- Pharmacol*). Recently, it was shown that ajone can induce apoptosis in the human keratinocyte cell line HaCat and has a diminishing on BCC in vivo by down–regulating the expression of the apoptosis- suppressing protein Bcl-2 (*Tilli et al, 2003, Arch Dermatol-Res*). A SHH antagonist, the Veratrum alkaloid cyclopamine (11-deoxojervine) can be used to treat BCC (*Taipale et al, 2000, Nature*). Interestingly cyclopamine binds directly to Smoothened, which explains its activity in tumours characterised by activated SHH pathways (*Chen et al, 2002, Proc Natl Acad Sci USA*). Interestingly its application to the surface of the tumour resulted not only in the rapid induction of apoptosis but also influenced the differentiation status 7 of 7 tumours (*Tas et al, 2004, Eur J Dermatol*)

5.2 Modulation of differentiation

Systemic retinoids are frequently used for chemoprevention of cutaneous malignancies in organ transplant recipients (Chen *et al, 2005,* Br J Dermatol.). Retinoids (vitamin A metabolites and analogues) have been shown to have suppressive effects on tumour promotion when administered in high doses, and the mechanism appears to be associated with modulation of growth, differentiation and apoptosis (*Lotan et al, 1996, Faseb J*). Retinoids are most effective in patients with multiple previous non-melanoma skin cancers (Kovach *et al, 2005,*Clin Transplant.) Low-dose systemic retinoids significantly reduce SCC development in organ transplant recipients for the first 3 years of treatment, and this effect may be sustained for at least 8 years (Harwood *et al, 2005,*Arch Dermatol.) It has been shown that retinoic acid is effective in inhibiting telomerase activity in HSC-1 human cutaneous squamous cell carcinoma cells (Kunisada *et al, 2005,*Br J Dermatol.).

5.3 Immunomodulation

Because BCCs often elicit a strong inflammatory response, recent studies have sought to evaluate the effects of immunomodulatory compounds. On of the most promising is imiquimod, a Toll- like receptor 7/8 agonist that enhances the endogenous cytokine response (INF- α, IL-10, TNF-α) among others stimulating the T- helper 1 - mediated inflammatory responses.

6. Conclusions/ future directions

In the past decade, significant progress has been made, in understanding the molecular genetics of NMSC and the molecular pathways involving tumour suppressor genes and oncogenes. Research into immune response to p53 had led to promising therapeutic potential. p53-specific cytotoxic T lymphocytes capable of mediating protective immunity to tumours have been generated in murine models (*Black et al, 2003,*Clin Exp Immunol.). Adoptive transfer of p53 specific cytotoxic T lymphocytes generated in p53-/- mice confers immunity on the recipient to p53 overexpressing murine tumour (Vierboom *et al, 1997,*J Exp Med.). As p53 is over expressed in cutaneous SCC, vaccination against p53 is a logical approach to induce tumour reactive immunity (*Black et al , 2003,*Clin Exp Immunol.) Vaccines used to induce p53 specific immune responses in mice have included, Canary pox virus vectors (*Roth et al, 1996,*Proc Natl Acad Sci U S A.), peptide pulsed dendritic cells (Mayordomo *et al, 1996,* J Exp Med.), recombinant adenovirus transduced dendritic cells (Ishida *et al, 1999,* Clin Exp Immunol., Nikitina , *2002,*Gene Ther.*)*, recombinant DNA, (Petersen *et al, 1999,*Cancer Lett.) recombinant vaccinia virus (Chen *et al, 2000,* Cancer Gene Ther.) and pulsed human monocyte-derived dendritic cells (Tokunaga *et al, 2005,*Clin Cancer Res.). However, besides p53, many genes are involved in the pathogenesis of SCC and an understanding into the genomic of SCC is far from complete. It is very likely that new genetic and molecular pathways for SCC genesis will unravel in the future, hopefully leading to novel therapies.

Clearly exposure to UVR is an important initiating factor in skin cancer, though the exact relationship between BCC risk and nature, extent and timing of exposure remains poorly understood. More recently, the influence of genetic factors influencing BCC susceptibility has been an area of intense interest with many genes having a similar impact as traditional risk factors such as skin type. Data so far suggests that risk of sporadic BCC is likely to result from the combined effect of many genes (defining distinct areas of biochemical activity) each with a relatively weak individual contribution, rather than a small number of highly influential genes.

Presumably, the effect of disruption of these biochemical activities will result in dysregulation of expression of key TSG or oncogenes. In this regard, the function of the hedgehog signalling pathway appears critical in BCC development. Though the *PTCH* gene has been suggested to be the 'gatekeeper' for BCC development, future studies will need to address the role of other members of this pathway. There are no studies to date focusing on the interaction between susceptibility genes and mutational events in TSG in BCC; this may represent a way forward.

7. References

[1] Ahmadian A, Ren ZP, Williams C et al. Genetic instability in the 9q22.3 region is a late event in the development of squamous cell carcinoma. *Oncogene.* 1998 Oct 8;17(14):1837-43.

[2] Albright SD 3rd. Treatment of skin cancer using multiple modalities. *J Am Acad Dermatol.* 1982 Aug;7(2):143-71

[3] Apitz-Castro R, Ledezma E, Escalante J et al. Reversible prevention of platelet activation by (E,Z)-4,5,9-trithiadodeca-1,6,11-triene 9-oxide (ajoene) in dogs under extracorporeal circulation. *Arzneimittelforschung.* 1988 Jul;38(7):901-4.

[4] Arbiser JL, Fine JD, Murrell D et al. Basic fibroblast growth factor: a missing link between collagen VII, increased collagenase, and squamous cell carcinoma in recessive dystrophic epidermolysis bullosa. *Mol Med.* 1998 Mar;4(3):191-5.

[5] Arbiser JL, Fan CY, Su X et al.Involvement of p53 and p16 tumor suppressor genes in recessive dystrophic epidermolysis bullosa-associated squamous cell carcinoma. *J Invest Dermatol.* 2004 Oct;123(4):788-90.

[6] Asplund A, Gustafsson AC, Wikonkal NM et al. PTCH codon 1315 polymorphism and risk for nonmelanoma skin cancer. *Br J Dermatol.* 2005 May;152(5):868-73.

[7] Aszterbaum M, Rothman A, Johnson RL et al. Identification of mutations in the human PATCHED gene in sporadic basal cell carcinomas and in patients with the basal cell nevus syndrome. *J Invest Dermatol.* 1998 Jun;110(6):885-8.

[8] AszterbaumM, EpsteinJ, OroA etal. Ultraviolet and ionizing radiation enhance the growth of BCCs and trichoblastomas in patched heterozygous knockout mice. *Nat Med.* 1999 Nov;5(11):1285-91.

[9] Auepemkiate S, Boonyaphiphat P, Thongsuksai P p53 expression related to the aggressive infiltrative histopathological feature of basal cell carcinoma. *Histopathology.* 2002 Jun;40(6):568-73.

[10] Avgerinou G, Nicolis G, Vareltzidis A, Stratigos J. The dermal cellular infiltrate and cell-mediated immunity in skin carcinomas. *Dermatologica.* 1985; 71(4):238- 42.

[11] Barrett WL, First MR, Aron BS et al. Clinical course of malignancies in renal transplant recipients. *Cancer.* 1993 Oct 1;72(7):2186-9.

[12] Barr BB, Benton EC, McLaren K. Papillomavirus infection and skin cancer in renal allograft recipients . *Lancet.* 1989 Jul 22;2(8656):224-5.

[13] Bale AE, Yu KP The hedgehog pathway and basal cell carcinomas *Hum Mol Genet.* 2001 Apr;10(7):757-62.

[14] Bavinck JN, Kootte AM, van der Woude F et al. HLA-A11-associated resistance to skin cancer in renal-transplant patients. *N Engl J Med.* 1990 Nov 8;323(19):1350

[15] Bavinck JN, Bastiaens MT, Marugg ME et al. Further evidence for an association of HLA-DR7 with basal cell carcinoma on the tropical island of Saba. *Arch Dermatol.* 2000 Aug;136(8):1019-22.

[16] Bavinck JN, De Boer A, Vermeer BJ et al. Sunlight, keratotic skin lesions and skin cancer in renal transplant recipients. *Br J Dermatol.* 1993 Sep; 129(3): 242-9.

[17] Berg RJ, van Kranen HJ, Rebel HG et al. Early p53 alterations in mouse skin carcinogenesis by UVB radiation: immunohistochemical detection of mutant p53 protein in clusters of preneoplastic epidermal cells. *Proc Natl Acad Sci U S A.* 1996 Jan 9;93(1):274-8.

[18] Benacerraf B. Role of MHC gene products in immune regulation. *Science.*1981Jun12;212(4500):1229-38

[19] Betti R, Tolomio E, Vergani R, Crosti C. Squamous epithelial carcinoma as a complication of lupus vulgaris. *Hautarzt.* 2002 Feb;53(2):118-20.

[20] Black AP, Ogg GSThe role of p53 in the immunobiology of cutaneous squamous cell carcinoma. *Clin Exp Immunol.* 2003 Jun;132(3):379-84.

[21] Bodak N, Queille S, Avril M F et al. High levels of patched gene mutations in basal-cell carcinomas from patients with xeroderma pigmentosum. *Proc Natl Acad Sci U S A.* 1999 Apr 27;96(9):5117-22.

[22] Boorstein RJ, Chiu LN, Teebor GW. Phylogenetic evidence of a role for 5-hydroxymethyluracil-DNA glycosylase in the maintenance of 5-methylcytosine in DNA. *Nucleic Acids Res.* 1989 Oct 11;17(19):7653-61.

[23] Bosch FX, Lorincz A, Munoz NThe causal relation between human papillomavirus and cervical cancer. *J Clin Pathol.* 2002 Apr;55(4):244-65.

[24] Bouwes Bavinck JN, Vermeer BJ, van der Woude FJ et al. Relation between skin cancer and HLA antigens in renal-transplant recipients. *N Engl J Med.* 1991 Sep 19;325(12):843-8.

[25] Bouwes Bavinck JN. Epidemiological aspects of immunosuppression: role of exposure to sunlight and human papillomavirus on the development of skin cancer. *Hum Exp Toxicol.* 1995 Jan;14(1):98.

[26] Bouwes Bavinck JN, Hardie DR, Green A et al. The risk of skin cancer in renal transplant recipients in Queensland, Australia. A follow-up study. *Transplantation.* 1996 Mar 15; 61(5):715-21.

[27] Bouwes-Bavinck JN, Claas FHJ, Hardie DR et al. Relation between HLA antigens and skin cancer in renal transplant recipients in Queensland. *Australia J Invest Dermatol* 1997;108:708-11.

[28] Bouwes Bavinck JN, Stark S, Petridis AK et al.The presence of antibodies against virus-like particles of epidermodysplasia verruciformis-associated humanpapillomavirus type 8 in patients with actinic keratoses. *Br J Dermatol.* 2000 Jan;142(1):103-9.

[29] Box NF, Duffy DL, Irving RE et al. Melanocortin-1 receptor genotype is a risk factor for basal and squamous cell carcinoma. *J Invest Dermatol.* 2001 Feb;116(2):224-9.

[30] Brash DE, Rudolph JA, Simon JA et al. A role for sunlight in skin cancer: UV- induced p53 mutations in squamous cell carcinoma. *Proc Natl Acad Sci U S A.* 1991 Nov 15;88(22):10124-8.

[31] Brash D E, Ponten J. Skin precancer. *Cancer Surv.*1998; 32:69-113.

[32] Brown VL, Harwood CA, Crook T et al. p16INK4a and p14ARF tumor suppressor genes are commonly inactivated in cutaneous squamous cell carcinoma. *J Invest Dermatol.* 2004 May;122(5):1284-92.

[33] Buechner S A, Wernli M, Harr T et al. Regression of basal cell carcinoma by intralesional interferon-alpha treatment is mediated by CD95 (Apo-1/Fas)-CD95 ligand-induced suicide. *J Clin Invest.* 1997 Dec 1;100(11):2691-6.

[34] Cabrera T, Garrido V, Concha A et al. HLA molecules in basal cell carcinoma of the skin.*Immunobiology.*1992Sep;185(5):440-52.

[35] Carless MA, Lea RA, Curran JE et al. The GSTM1 null genotype confers an increased risk for solar keratosis development in an Australian Caucasian population.*J Invest Dermatol.* 2002 Dec;119(6):1373-8.

[36] Caspari T. How to activate p53.*Curr Biol.* 2000 Apr 20;10(8):R315-7

[37] Chen JK, Taipale J, Cooper MK et al. Inhibition of Hedgehog signaling by direct binding of cyclopamine to Smoothened. *Genes Dev.* 2002 Nov 1;16(21):2743-8.

[38] Chen B, Timiryasova TM, Andres ML et al. Evaluation of combined vaccinia virus-mediated antitumor gene therapy with p53, IL-2, and IL-12 in a glioma model. *Cancer Gene Ther.* 2000 Nov;7(11):1437-47.

[39] Chen K, Craig JC, Shumack S. Oral retinoids for the prevention of skin cancers in solid organ transplant recipients: a systematic review of randomized controlled trials. *Br J Dermatol.* 2005 Mar;152(3):518-23.

[40] Cleaver JE. Xeroderma pigmentosum: a human disease in which an initial stage of DNA repair is defective. *Proc Natl Acad Sci USA* 1969; 63: 428-35.

[41] Coulter LK, Wolber R, Tron VA. Site-specific comparison of p53immunostaining in squamous cell carcinomas. *Hum Pathol.* 1995 May;26(5): 531-3.

[42] Crispian S. The oral cavity and lips. In Rooks textbook of Dermatology,7th Edition. Burns T, Breathnach S, Cox N, Griffiths C. Blackwell publishing.66.87

[43] Czarnecki D, Lewis A, Nicholson I et al.HLA-DR1 is not a sign of poor prognosis for the development of multiple basal cell carcinomas. *J Am Acad Dermatol.* 1992 May;26(5 Pt 1):717-9.

[44] Czarnecki D, Nicholson I, Tait B, Nash C. HLA DR4 is associated with the development of multiple basal cell carcinomas and malignant melanoma. *Dermatology.* 1993;187(1):16-8.

[45] Dahmane N, Lee J, Robins P et al. Activation of the transcription factor Gli1 and the Sonic hedgehog signalling pathway in skin tumours. *Nature.* 1997 Oct 23;389 (6653):876-81.

[46] Dantal J, Hourmant M, Cantarovich D et al. Effect of long-term immunosuppression in kidney-graft recipients on cancer incidence: randomised comparison of two cyclosporin regimens. *Lancet* 1998 Feb 28;351(9103):623-8.

[47] Dausset J, Colombani J, Hors J. Major Histocompatibility complex and cancer, with special reference to human family tumours. (Hodgkin's disease and other malignancies) *Cancer Surv* 1982;1: 119-47.

[48] de Berker D, Ibbotson S, Simpson NB et al. Reduced experimental contact sensitivity in squamous cell but not basal cell carcinomas of skin. *Lancet.* 1995Feb18;345(8947):425-6.

[49] Dellavalle RP, Walsh P, Marchbank A et al. CUSP/p63 expression in basal cell carcinoma. *Exp Dermatol.* 2002 Jun;11(3):203-8.

[50] Demirkan NC, Colakoglu N, Duzcan E. Value of p53 protein in biological behavior of basal cell carcinoma and in normal epithelia adjacent to carcinomas. *Pathol Oncol Res.* 2000;6(4):272-4.

[51] Di Como CJ, Urist MJ, Babayan I. p63 expression profiles in human normal and tumor tissues. *Clin Cancer Res.* 2002 Feb;8(2):494-501.

[52] Dirsch VM, Gerbes AL, Vollmar AM.. Ajoene, a compound of garlic, induces apoptosis in human promyeloleukemic cells, accompanied by generation of reactive oxygen species and activation of nuclear factor kappa *B. Mol Pharmacol.* 1998Mar;53(3):402-7.

[53] Dowell SP, Wilson PO, Derias NW et al. Clinical utility of the immunocytochemical detection of p53 protein in cytological specimens. *Cancer Res.* 1994 Jun 1;54(11):2914-8

[54] Duman-Scheel M, Weng L, Xin S et al. Hedgehog regulates cell growth and proliferation by inducing Cyclin D and Cyclin E. Nature. 2002 May 16;417(6886):299-304.

[55] Eklund LK, Lindstrom E, Unden AB et al. Mutation analysis of the human homologue of Drosophila patched and the xeroderma pigmentosum complementation group A genes in squamous cell carcinomas of the skin. *Mol Carcinog.* 1998 Feb;21(2):87-92.

[56] Elbel M, Carl S, Spaderna S, Iftner T A comparative analysis of the interactions of the E6 proteins from cutaneous and genital papillomaviruses with p53 and E6AP in correlation to their transforming potential. *Virology.* 1997 Dec 8;239 (1):132-49.

[57] Ellis NA, Groden J, Ye TZ et al . The Bloom's syndrome gene product is homologous to RecQ helicases. Cell. 1995 Nov 17;83(4):655-66

[58] Euvrard S, Kanitakis J, Pouteil-Noble C. Comparative epidemiologic study of premalignant and malignant epithelial cutaneous lesions developing after kidney and heart transplantation.*J Am Acad Dermatol.* 1995 Aug;33(2 Pt 1):222-9.

[59] Fan H, Oro AE, Scott MP et al. Induction of basal cell carcinoma features in transgenic human skin expressing Sonic Hedgehog. *Nat Med.* 1997 Jul;3(7):788-92.

[60] FanH, KhavariPA Sonic hedgehog opposes epithelial cell cycle arrest. *Cell Biol.*1999 Oct 4;147(1):71-6.

[61] Feltkamp MC, Broer R, di Summa FM et al. Seroreactivity to epidermodysplasia verruciformis-related human papillomavirus types is associated with nonmelanoma skin cancer. *Cancer Res.* 2003 May 15;63(10):2695-700.

[62] Fisher DE Apoptosis in cancer therapy: crossing the threshold. *Cell.* 1994 Aug 26;78(4):539-42.

[63] Forstrum L. Carcinomatous changes in lupus vulgaris. *Ann Clin Res* 1969;1:213.

[64] Franceschi S, Dal Maso L, Arniani S et al.Risk of cancer other than Kaposi's sarcoma and non-Hodgkin's lymphoma in persons with AIDS in Italy. Cancer and AIDS Registry Linkage Study. *Br J Cancer.* 1998 Oct;78(7):966-70.

[65] Gailani MR, Leffell DJ, Ziegler AJ et al. Relationship between sunlight exposure and a key genetic alteration in basal cell carcinoma. *Natl Cancer Inst.* 1996 Mar 20;88(6):349-54.

[66] Gailani MR, Stahle-Backdahl M, Leffell DJ et al. The role of the human homologue of Drosophila patched in sporadic basal cell carcinomas. *Nat Genet.* 1996 Sep;14(1):78-81.

[67] GallowayDA,McDougallJK. Human papillomaviruses and carcinomas. *Adv Virus Res.* 1989;37:125-71.

[68] Garcia-PlataD,MozosE,SierraMA et al. HLA expression in basal cell carcinomas. *Invasion Metastasis.* 1991;11(3):166-73.

[69] Grachtchouk M, Mo R, Yu S et al. Basal cell carcinomas in mice overexpressing Gli2 in skin. *Nat Genet.* 2000 Mar;24(3):216-7.

[70] Granstein RD.Cytokines and photocarcinogenesis. *Photochem Photobiol.* 1996 Apr;63(4):390-4.

[71] Griffiths HR, Mistry P, Herbert KE, Lunec J. Molecular and cellular effects of ultraviolet light-induced genotoxicity. *Crit Rev Clin Lab Sci.* 1998 Jun;35(3): 89-237.

[72] Hahn H, Wicking C, Zaphiropoulous PG et al. Mutations of the human homolog of Drosophila patched in the nevoid basal cell carcinoma syndrome. *Cell.* 1996 Jun 14;85(6):841-51.
[73] Hajeer A H, Lear J T, Ollier WE et al. Preliminary evidence of an association of tumour necrosis factor microsatellites with increased risk of multiple basal cell carcinomas.*BrJDermatol.*2000Mar;142(3):441-5.
[74] Hall PA, McKee PH, Menage HD et al. High levels of p53 protein in UV- irradiated normal humans kin. *Oncogene.* 1993 Jan;8(1):203-7.
[75] Hall J, English DR, Artuso M, et al. DNA repair capacity as a risk factor for non-melanocytic skin cancer-a molecular epidemiology study. *Int J Cancer* 1994; 58: 179-84.
[76] Han J, Colditz GA, Liu JS, Hunter DJ. Genetic variation in XPD, sun exposure, and risk of skin cancer. *Cancer Epidemiol Biomarkers Prev.* 2005 Jun;14(6):1539-44
[77] Han J, Colditz GA, Samson LD, Hunter DJ. Polymorphisms in DNA double- strand break repair genes and skin cancer risk. *Cancer Res.* 2004 May 1;64(9):3009-13.
[78] Han J, Hankinson SE, Colditz GA, Hunter DJ. Genetic variation in XRCC1, sun exposure, and risk of skin cancer.*Br J Cancer.* 2004 Oct 18;91(8):1604-9.
[79] Hartevelt MM, Bavinck JN, Kootte AM et al. Incidence of skin cancer after renal transplantation in The Netherlands. *Transplantation.* 1990 Mar;49(3):506-9.
[80] Harwood CA, Proby CM. Human papillomaviruses and non-melanoma skin cancer. *Curr Opin Infect Dis.* 2002 Apr;15(2):101-14.
[81] Harwood CA, Leedham-Green M, Leigh IM, Proby CM.Low-dose retinoids in the prevention of cutaneous squamous cell carcinomas in organ transplant recipients: a 16-year retrospective study. *Arch Dermatol.* 2005 Apr;141(4):456- 64.
[82] Haupt Y, Maya R, Kazaz A et al. Mdm2 promotes the rapid degradation of p53.*Nature.* 1997 May 15;387(6630):296-9.
[83] Hayes J D, Pulford DJ .The glutathione S-transferase supergene family: regulation of GST and the contribution of the isoenzymes to cancer chemoprotection and drug resistance. *Crit Rev Biochem Mol Biol.* 1995;30(6):445-600.
[84] Heagerty A H, Fitzgerald D, Smith A. Glutathione S-transferase GSTM1 phenotypes and protection against cutaneous tumours. *Lancet.* 1994Jan29; 343(8892):266-8.
[85] Heagerty A, Smith A, English J et al. Susceptibility to multiple cutaneous basal cell carcinomas: significant interactions between glutathione S-transferase GSTM1 genotypes, skin type and male gender. *Br J Cancer.* 1996 Jan;73(1):44-8
[86] Hoffman EJ, Cancer and the search for selective biochemical inhibitors. Boca Raton, FL, CRC Press, 1999.
[87] Hollstein M, Sidransky D, Vogelstein B et al. p53 mutations in human cancers. *Science.* 1991 Jul 5;253(5015):49-53.
[88] Holme SA, Malinovszky K, Roberts DL Changing trends in non-melanoma skin cancer in South Wales, 1988-98. Br J Dermatol. 2000 Dec;143(6):1224-9.
[89] Huang Z. Bcl-2 family proteins as targets for anticancer drug design. *Oncogene.* 2000 Dec 27;19(56):6627-31.

[90] Ishida T, Chada S, Stipanov M et al. Dendritic cells transduced with wild-type p53 gene elicit potent anti-tumour immune responses. *Clin Exp Immunol.* 1999 Aug;117(2):244-51
[91] Jackson S, Harwood C, Thomas M et al. Role of Bak in UV-induced apoptosis in skin cancer and abrogation by HPV E6 proteins. *Genes Dev.* 2000 Dec 1;14(23):3065-73.
[92] Jee S H, Shen S C, Tseng C R et al. Curcumin induces a p53-dependent apoptosis in humanbasalcellcarcinomacells. *J Invest Dermatol.* 1998 Oct;111(4):656-61.
[93] Jee SH, Shen SC, Chiu HC et al. Overexpression of interleukin-6 in human basal cell carcinoma cell lines increases anti-apoptotic activity and tumorigenic potency. *Oncogene.* 2001 Jan 11;20(2):198-208.
[94] Jensen P, Hansen S, Moller BJ et al . Skin cancer in kidney and heart transplant recipients and different long-term immunosuppressive therapy regimens. *Am Acad Dermatol* 1999 Feb;40(2 Pt 1):177-86
[95] Johnson RL, Rothman AL, Xie J et al. Human homolog of patched, a candidate gene for the basal cell nevus syndrome. *Science.* 1996 Jun 14;272(5268):1668-71.
[96] Jonason AS, Kunala S, Price GJ et al. Frequent clones of p53-mutated keratinocytes in normal human skin. *Proc Natl Acad Sci U S A.* 1996 Nov 26;93(24):14025-9.
[97] Kalka K, Merk H, Mukhtar H et al. Photodynamic therapy in dermatology.*J Am Acad Dermatol.* 2000 Mar;42(3):389-413; quiz 414-6.
[98] Kallassy M, Toftgard R, Ueda M et al. Patched (ptch)-associated preferential expression of smoothened (smoh) in human basal cell carcinoma of the skin. *Cancer Res.* 1997 Nov 1;57(21):4731-5
[99] Karagas MR, Greenberg ER. Unresolved issues in the epidemiology of basal cell and squamous cell skin cancer. In: Skin cancer: Mechanisms and human relevance. (Mukhtar H., ed.) Boca Raton, Florida: CRC Press, 1995: 79-86.
[100] Kaplan RP. Cancer complicating chronic ulcerative and scarring mucocutaneous disorders. *Adv Derm* 1987;2: 19-46.
[101] Kastan MB, Onyekwere O, Sidransky D et al. Participation of p53 protein in the cellular response to DNA damage. *Cancer Res.* 1991 Dec 1;51(23 Pt 1):6304-11.
[102] Katayama H, Sasai K, Kawai H et al. Phosphorylation by aurora kinase A induces Mdm2-mediated destabilization and inhibition of p53. *Nat Genet.* 2004 Jan;36(1):55-62.
[103] Kerb R, Brockmoller J, Reum T et al. Deficiency of glutathione S-transferases T1 and M1 as heritable factors of increased cutaneous UV sensitivity. *J Invest Dermatol.* 1997 Feb;108(2):229-32.
[104] Kim MY, Park HJ, Baek SC et al. Mutations of the p53 and PTCH gene in basal cell carcinomas: UV mutation signature and strand bias. *J Dermatol Sci.* 2002 May;29(1):1-9.
[105] Kitao S, Lindor NM, Shiratori M et al. Rothmund-thomson syndrome responsible gene, RECQL4: genomic structure and products. *Genomics* 1999 Nov 1;61(3):268-76.
[106] Knight SW, Heiss NS, Vulliamy TJ et al. X-linked dyskeratosis congenita is predominantly caused by missense mutations in the DKC1 gene. *Am J Hum Genet.* 1999 Jul;65(1):50-8.

[107] Knudson A G Jr. Hereditary cancer, oncogenes, and antioncogenes. *Cancer Res.* 1985Apr;45(4):1437-43.

[108] Koehl GE, Andrassy J, Guba M et al. Rapamycin protects allografts from rejection while simultaneously attacking tumors in immunosuppressed mice. *Transplantation.* 2004 May 15;77(9):1319-26.

[109] Koike C, Mizutani T, Ito T, Shimizu Y. Introduction of wild-type patched gene suppresses the oncogenic potential of human squamous cell carcinoma cell lines including A431. *Oncogene.* 2002 Apr 18;21(17):2670-8.

[110] Kovach BT, Sams HH, Stasko T. Systemic strategies for chemoprevention of skin cancers in transplant recipients. *Clin Transplant.* 2005 Dec;19(6):726-34.

[111] Kreimer-Erlacher H, Seidl H, Back B, Kerl H, Wolf P. High mutation frequency at Ha-ras exons 1-4 in squamous cell carcinomas from PUVA-treated psoriasis patients. *Photochem Photobiol.* 2001 Aug;74(2):323-30.

[112] Kricker A, Armstrong BK, English DR, Heenan PJ. Does intermittent sun exposure cause basal cell carcinoma? A case-control study in Western Australia. *Int J Cancer* 1995; 60: 489-94.

[113] Kricker A, Armstrong BK, English DR, Heenan PJ. A dose-response curve for sun exposure and basal cell carcinoma. *Int J Cancer.* 1995 Feb ;60(4):482- 8.

[114] Kripke ML. Ultraviolet radiation and immunology: something new under the sun--presidentialaddress. *Cancer Res.* 1994 Dec 1;54(23):6102-5.

[115] Kubbutat MH, Jones SN, Vousden KH. Regulation of p53 stability by Mdm2. *Nature.* 1997 May 15;387(6630):299-303.

[116] Kunisada M, Budiyanto A, Bito T et al. Retinoic acid suppresses telomerase activity in HSC-1 human cutaneous squamous cell carcinoma. *Br J Dermatol.* 2005 Mar;152(3):435-43.

[117] Kutler DI, Wreesmann VB, Goberdhan A et al. Human papillomavirus DNA and p53 polymorphisms in squamous cell carcinomas from Fanconi anemia patients. *J Natl Cancer Inst.* 2003 Nov 19;95(22):1718-21.

[118] Lavker RM, Miller SJ, Sun TT. Epithelial stem cells, hair follicles, and tumor formation. *Recent Results Cancer Res.* 1993;128:31-43.

[119] Lear JT, Heagerty AH, Smith A et al.Multiple cutaneous basal cell carcinomas: glutathione S-transferase (GSTM1, GSTT1) and cytochrome P450 (CYP2D6, CYP1A1) polymorphisms influence tumour numbers and accrual. *Carcinogenesis.* 1996 Sep;17(9):1891-6.

[120] Lear JT, Smith AG, Heagerty AH. et al. Truncal site and detoxifying enzyme polymorphisms significantly reduce time to presentation of further primary cutaneous basal cell carcinoma. *Carcinogenesis.*1997Aug;18(8):1499-503.

[121] Lear JT, Smith AG, Strange RC, Fryer AA Detoxifying enzyme genotypes and susceptibility to cutaneous malignancy. *Br J Dermatol.* 2000 Jan;142(1):8-15.

[122] Leite JL, Stolf HO, Reis NA, Ward LS. Human herpesvirus type 6 and type 1 infection increases susceptibility to nonmelanoma skin tumors. *Cancer Lett.* 2005 Jun 28;224(2):213-9.

[123] Liang SB, Ohtsuki Y, Furihata M et al.Sun-exposure- and aging-dependent p53 protein accumulation results in growth advantage for tumour cells in carcinogenesis of nonmelanocytic skin cancer. *Virchows Arch.* 1999 Mar;434(3):193-9.

[124] Liefer KM, Koster MI, Wang XJ et al. Down-regulation of p63 is required for epidermal UV-B-induced apoptosis. *Cancer Res.* 2000 Aug 1;60(15):4016-20.

[125] Little NA, Jochemsen AG.p63. *Int J Biochem Cell Biol.* 2002 Jan;34(1):6-9.

[126] Lobo D V, Chu P, Grekin R C et al. Nonmelanoma skin cancers and infection with the human immunodeficiency virus.*ArchDermatol.*1992May; 128(5):623-7.

[127] Lotan R. Retinoids in cancer chemoprevention. *Faseb J.* 1996 Jul;10(9):1031-9

[128] Lookingbill DP, Lookingbill GL, Leppard B. Actinic damage and skin cancer in albinos in northern Tanzania: findings in 164 patients enrolled in an outreach skin care program. *J Am Acad Dermatol.* 1995 Apr;32(4):653-8.

[129] Lu YP, Lou YR, Xie JG et al. Inhibitory effect of black tea on the growth of established skin tumors in mice: effects on tumor size, apoptosis, mitosis and bromodeoxyuridine incorporation into DNA. *Carcinogenesis.* 1997 Nov;18(11):2163-9.

[130] Madariaga J, Fromowitz F, Phillips M.Squamous cell carcinoma in congenital ichthyosis with deafness and keratitis. A case report and review of the literature. *Cancer.* 1986 May 15;57(10):2026-9.

[131] Majewski S, Jablonska S Epidermodysplasia verruciformis as a model of human papillomavirus-induced genetic cancer of the skin. *Arch Dermatol.* 1995 Nov;131(11):1312-8.

[132] Maki CG, Huibregtse JM, Howley PM.In vivo ubiquitination and proteasome-mediated degradation of p53(1).*Cancer Res.* 1996 Jun 1;56(11):2649-54.

[133] Malkin D, Li FP, Strong LC et al . Germ line p53 mutations in a familial syndrome of breast cancer, sarcomas, and other neoplasms. *Science.* 1990 Nov 30;250(4985):1233-8.

[134] Mallipeddi R, Wessagowit V, South AP et al. Reduced expression of insulin-like growth factor-binding protein-3 (IGFBP-3) in Squamous cell carcinoma complicating recessive dystrophic epidermolysis bullosa. *J Invest Dermatol.* 2004 May;122(5):1302-9.

[135] Marks R, Foley P, Goodman G et al. Spontaneous remission of solar keratoses: the case for conservative management. *Br J Dermatol.* 1986 Dec;115(6):649-55.

[136] Masini C, Fuchs PG, Gabrielli F et al. Evidence for the association of human papillomavirus infection and cutaneous squamous cell carcinoma in immunocompetent individuals. *Arch Dermatol.* 2003 Jul;139(7):890-4.

[137] Mayordomo JI, Loftus DJ, Sakamoto H et al. Therapy of murine tumors with p53 wild-type and mutant sequence peptide-based vaccines. *J Exp Med.* 1996 Apr 1;183(4):1357-65.

[138] McGregor JM, Proby CM. Skin cancer in transplant recipients. *Lancet.* 1995 Oct 7;346(8980):964-5.

[139] McLelland J, Rees A, Williams G et al. The incidence of immunosuppression- related skin disease in long-term transplant patients. *Transplantation.* 1988 Dec;46(6):871-4.

[140] Miller BH, Shavin JS, Cognetta A Nonsurgical treatment of basal cell carcinomas with intralesional 5-fluorouracil/epinephrine injectable gel. *J Am Acad Dermatol.* 1997 Jan;36(1):72-7.

[141] Miller SJ, Sun TT, Lavker RM. Hair follicles, stem cells, and skin cancer. *J Invest Dermatol.*1993Mar; 100(3):288S-294S.

[142] Mills AA, Zheng B, Wang X J et al. p63 is a p53 homologue required for limb and epidermal morphogenesis. *Nature.* 1999 Apr 22;398(6729):708-13.

[143] Moscow JA, Townsend AJ, Goldsmith M et al. Isolation of the human anionic glutathione S-transferase cDNA and the relation of its gene expression to estrogen-receptor content in primary breast cancer .*Proc Natl Acad Sci U S A.* 1988 Sep;85(17):6518-22.

[144] Myskowski P L, Safai B, Good R A. Decreased lymphocyte blastogenic responses in patients with multiple basal cellcarcinoma. *J Am Acad Dermatol.* 1981 Jun;4(6):711-4.

[145] Nakaseko H, Kobayashi M, Akita Y et al. Histological changes and involvement of apoptosis after photodynamic therapy for actinic keratoses. *Br J Dermatol.* 2003, Jan;148(1):122-7.

[146] Nakazawa H, English D, Randell PLProc et al. UV and skin cancer: specific p53 gene mutation in normal skin as a biologically relevant exposure measurement. *Natl Acad Sci U S A.* 1994 Jan 4;91(1):360-4.

[147] Nataraj AJ, Trent JC 2nd, Ananthaswamy HN. p53 gene mutations and photocarcinogenesis. *Photochem Photobiol.* 1995 Aug;62(2):218-30

[148] Nelson HH, Christensen B, Karagas MR. The XPC poly-AT polymorphism in non-melanoma skin cancer. *Cancer Lett.* 2005 May 26;222(2):205-9.

[149] Nikitina EY, Chada S, Muro-Cacho C et al An effective immunization and cancer treatment with activated dendritic cells transduced with full-length wild-type p53. *Gene Ther.* 2002 Mar;9(5):345-52.

[150] Nilsson M, Unden AB, Krause D et al. Induction of basal cell carcinomas and trichoepitheliomas in mice overexpressing GLI-1.*Proc Natl Acad Sci U S A.* 2000 Mar 28;97(7):3438-43.

[151] O'Donovan P, Perrett CM, Zhang X et al. Azathioprine and UVA light generate mutagenic oxidative DNA damage. *Science.* 2005 Sep 16;309 (5742):1871-4.

[152] Ondrus D, Pribylincova V, Breza J et al. The incidence of tumours in renal transplant recipients with long-term immunosuppressive therapy. *Int Urol Nephrol.* 1999;31(4):417-22

[153] Ong CS, Keogh AM, Kossard S et al. Skin cancer in Australian heart transplant recipients.*J Am Acad Dermatol.* 1999 Jan;40(1):27-34.

[154] Oro A E, Higgins K M, Hu Z et al. Basal cell carcinomas in mice overexpressing sonic hedgehog. *Science.* 1997 May 2;276(5313):817-21.

[155] Otley CC, Pittelkow MR. Skin cancer in liver transplant recipients. *Liver Transpl.* 2000 May;6(3):253-62.

[156] Pagano G, Zatterale A, Degan P et al. Multiple involvement of oxidative stress in Werner syndrome phenotype. *Biogerontology.* 2005;6(4):233-43.

[157] Pagano G, Zatterale A, Degan P et al et al. In vivo prooxidant state in Werner syndrome (WS): results from three WS patients and two WS heterozygotes. *Free Radic Res.* 2005 May;39(5):529-33.

[158] Park CB, Fukamachi K, Takasuka N et al. Rapid induction of skin and mammary tumors in human c-Ha-ras proto-oncogene transgenic rats by treatment with 7,12-dimethylbenz[a]anthracene followed by 12-O- tetradecanoylphorbol 13-acetate. *Cancer Sci.* 2004 Mar;95(3):205-10.

[159] Parsa R, Yang A, McKeon F et al. Association of p63 with proliferative potential in normal and neoplastic human keratinocytes. *J Invest Dermatol.* 1999 Dec;113(6):1099-105.

[160] Pemble S, Schroeder KR, Spencer SR et al. Human glutathione S-transferase theta (GSTT1): cDNA cloning and the characterization of a genetic polymorphism. *Biochem J.* 1994 May 15;300 (Pt 1):271-6.

[161] Penn I. The changing pattern of posttransplant malignancies. *Transplant Proc* 1991 Feb;23(1 Pt 2):1101-3.

[162] Penn I. Tumors after renal and cardiac transplantation. *Hematol Oncol Clin North Am.* 1993 Apr;7(2):431-45

[163] Peterkin GAG. Malignant change in erythema ab igne. *BMJ.* 1955; ii; 1599-602.

[164] Petersen TR, Bregenholta S, Pedersen LO et al.Human p53(264-272) HLA-A2 binding peptide is an immunodominant epitope in DNA-immunized HLA-A2 transgenic mice. *Cancer Lett.* 1999 Apr 1;137(2):183-91.

[165] Petkovic M, Dietschy T, Freire R et al. J Cell Sci. The human Rothmund- Thomson syndrome gene product, RECQL4, localizes to distinct nuclear foci that coincide with proteins involved in the maintenance of genome stability. *J Cell Sci.* 2005 Sep 15;118(Pt 18):4261-9

[166] Pfister H. Chapter 8: Human papillomavirus and skin cancer. *J Natl Cancer Inst Monogr.* 2003;(31):52-6.

[167] Pierceall WE, Goldberg LH, Tainsky MA et al. Ras gene mutation and amplification in human nonmelanoma skin cancers. *Mol Carcinog.* 991;4(3):196-202.

[168] Ping XL, Ratner D, Zhang H et al.PTCH mutations in squamous cell carcinoma of the skin.*J Invest Dermatol.* 2001 Apr;116(4):614-6.

[169] Piquero-Casals J, Okubo AY, Nico MM. Rothmund-thomson syndrome in three siblings and development of cutaneous squamous cell carcinoma. *Pediatr Dermatol.* 2002 Jul-Aug;19(4):312-6.

[170] Pritchard BN, Youngberg GA . Atypical mitotic figures in basal cell carcinoma. A review of 208 cases. *Am J Dermatopathol.* 1993 Dec;15(6):549-52.

[171] Purdie KJ, Pennington J, Proby CM et al. The promoter of a novel human papillomavirus (HPV77) associated with skin cancer displays UV responsiveness, which is mediated through a consensus p53 binding sequence. *EMBO J.* 1999 Oct 1;18(19):5359-69.

[172] Purdie KJ, Surentheran T, Sterling JC et al. Human papillomavirus gene expression in cutaneous squamous cell carcinomas from immunosuppressed and immunocompetent individuals. *J Invest Dermatol.* 2005 Jul;125(1):98-107.

[173] Quade BJ, Yang A, Wang Y et al. Expression of the p53 homologue p63 in early cervical neoplasia. *Gynecol Oncol.* 2001 Jan;80(1):24-9.

[174] Quinn AG, Sikkink S, Rees JL Basal cell carcinomas and squamous cell carcinomas of human skin show distinct patterns of chromosome loss. *Cancer Res.* 1994 Sep 1;54(17):4756-9.

[175] Rady P, Scinicariello F, Wagner RF Jr et al. p53 mutations in basal cell carcinomas. *Cancer Res.* 1992 Jul 1;52(13):3804-6.

[176] Ragni MV, Belle SH, Jaffe RA et al. Acquired immunodeficiency syndrome-associated non-Hodgkin's lymphomas and other malignancies in patients with hemophilia.*Blood.*1993Apr1;81(7):1889-97.

[177] Ramachandran S, Lear JT, Ramsay H, et al. Presentation with multiple cutaneous basal cell carcinomas: Association of glutathione S-transferase and cytochrome P450 genotypes with clinical phenotype. *Cancer Epidemiol Biomarkers Prev* 1999; 8: 61-7.

[178] Ramachandran S, Fryer AA, Lear JT, et al. Basal Cell Carcinoma: Tumor clustering is associated with increased accrual in high-risk subgroups. *Cancer* 2000; 89: 1012-8

[179] Ramachandran S, Fryer AA, Smith AG, et al. Cutaneous basal cell carcinomas: Distinct host factors are associated with the development of tumors on the trunk and head and neck. *Cancer* 2001; 92: 354-8.

[180] Raza H, Awasthi YC, Zaim MT et al.Glutathione S-transferases in human and rodent skin: multiple forms and species-specific expression. *J Invest Dermatol.* 1991Apr;96(4):463-7.

[181] Reis-Filho JS, Torio B, Albergaria A, Schmitt FC. p63 expression in normal skin and usual cutaneous carcinomas. *J Cutan Pathol.* 2002 Oct;29(9):517-23.

[182] Rodriguez-Villanueva J, McDonnell TJ. Induction of apoptotic cell death in non-melanoma skin cancer by interferon-alpha. *Int J Cancer.* 1995 Mar 29;61(1):110-4.

[183] Romkes M, Chern HD, Lesnick TG e al. Association of low CYP3A activity with p53 mutation and CYP2D6 activity with Rb mutation in human bladder cancer. *Carcinogenesis.* 1996 May;17(5):1057-62.

[184] Rompel R, Petres J, Kaupert K et al Human leukocyte antigens and multiple basal cell carcinomas. Recent Results. *Cancer Res.* 1995;139:297-302.

[185] Ronen D, Schwartz D, Teitz Y et al. Induction of HL-60 cells to undergo apoptosis is determined by high levels of wild-type p53 protein whereas differentiation of the cells is mediated by lower p53 levels. *Cell Growth Differ.*1996Jan;7(1):21-30.

[186] Rosenstein BS, Phelps RG, Weinstock MA et al. p53 mutations in basal cell carcinomas arising in routine users of sunscreens. *Photochem Photobiol.* 1999 Nov;70(5):798-806.

[187] Rosso S, Zanetti R, Martinez C, et al. The multicentre south European study "Helios" II: different sun exposure patterns in the aetiology of basal cell and squamous cell carcinomas of the skin. *Br J Cancer.* 1996; 73: 1447-54.

[188] Roth J, Dittmer D, Rea D et al. p53 as a target for cancer vaccines: recombinant canarypox virus vectors expressing p53 protect mice against lethal tumor cell challenge. *Proc Natl Acad Sci U S A.* 1996 May 14;93(10):4781-6.

[189] Ruhland A, de Villiers EMOpposite regulation of the HPV 20-URR and HPV 27-URR promoters by ultraviolet irradiation and cytokines. *Int J Cancer.* 2001 Mar 15;91(6):828-34.

[190] Ruiter DJ, Bergman W, Welvaart K et al. Immunohistochemical analysis of malignant melanomas and nevocellular nevi with monoclonal antibodies to distinct monomorphic determinants of HLA antigens. *Cancer Res.* 1984 Sep;44(9):3930-5.

[191] Salasche SJ. Epidemiology of actinic keratoses and squamous cell carcinoma. *J Am Acad Dermatol.* 2000 Jan;42(1 Pt 2):4-7.

[192] Sarhanis P, Redman C, Perrett C et al. Epithelial ovarian cancer: influence of polymorphism at the glutathione S-transferase GSTM1 and GSTT1 loci on p53 expression.*Br J Cancer.* 1996 Dec;74(11):1757-61.

[193] Shamanin V, zur Hausen H, Lavergne D J Natl. Human papillomavirus infections in nonmelanoma skin cancers from renal transplant recipients and nonimmunosuppressed patients. *Cancer Inst.* 1996 Jun 19;88(12):802-11.

[194] Shields JM, Pruitt K, McFall A et al. Understanding Ras: 'it ain't over 'til it's over'. *Trends Cell Biol.* 2000 Apr;10(4):147-54.

[195] Siliciano JD, Canman CE, Taya Y et al. DNA damage induces phosphorylation of the amino terminus of p53 .*Genes Dev.* 1997 Dec 15;11(24):3471-81.

[196] Sionov RV, Haupt Y. The cellular response to p53: the decision between life and death. *Oncogene.* 1999 Nov 1;18(45):6145-57.

[197] Sitz KV, Keppen M, Johnson DF Metastatic basal cell carcinoma in acquired immunodeficiency syndrome-elated complex. *JAMA.* 1987 Jan 16;257(3):340-3.

[198] Soufir N, Daya-Grosjean L, de La Salmoniere P et al. Association between INK4a-ARF and p53 mutations in skin carcinomas of xeroderma pigmentosum patients. *J Natl Cancer Inst.* 2000 Nov 15;92(22):1841-7.

[199] Soussi T. The p53 tumor suppressor gene: from molecular biology to clinical investigation. *Ann N Y Acad Sci.* 2000 Jun;910:121-37; discussion 137-9.

[200] Spencer JM, Kahn SM, Jiang W et al. Activated ras genes occur in human actinic keratoses, premalignant precursors to squamous cell carcinomas. *Arch Dermatol.* 1995 Jul;131(7):796-800.

[201] Sprong H, van der Sluijs P, van Meer G How proteins move lipids and lipids move proteins. *Nat Rev Mol Cell Biol.* 2001 Jul;2(7):504-13.

[202] Stanley M, Coleman N, Chambers M The host response to lesions induced by human papillomavirus. *Ciba Found Symp.* 1994;187:21-32; discussion 32-44.

[203] Steigleder GK. Metastasizing basalioma in AIDS. *Z Hautkr.* 1987 May 1;62(9):661.

[204] Stern RS, Lunder EJ. Risk of squamous cell carcinoma and methoxsalen (psoralen) and UV-A radiation (PUVA): a meta-analysis. *Arch Dermatol* 1998;134: 1582-5.

[205] Stone DM, Murone M, Luoh S et al. Characterization of the human suppressor of fused, a negative regulator of the zinc-finger transcription factor *Gli.J Cell Sci.* 1999 Dec;112 (Pt 23):4437-48.

[206] Storey A, Thomas M, Kalita A et al. *Nature.* Role of a p53 polymorphism in the development of human papillomavirus-associated cancer. *Nature,*1998 May 21;393(6682):229-34.

[207] Streilein JW. Sunlight and skin-associated lymphoid tissues (SALT): if UVB is the trigger and TNF alpha is its mediator, what is the message? *J Invest Dermatol.* 1993 Jan;100(1):47S-52S.

[208] Taipale J, Chen J K, Cooper M K et al. Effects of oncogenic mutations in Smoothened and Patched can be reversed by cyclopamine. *Nature.* 2000 Aug 31;406(6799):1005-9.

[209] TasS, Avci O, Induction of the differentiation and apoptosis of tumour cells in vivo with efficiency and selectivity. *Eur J Dermatol*2004;14:96-102

[210] Thissen MR, Schroeter C A, Neumann H A et al. Photodynamic therapy with delta-aminolaevulinic acid for nodular basal cell carcinomas using a prior debulking technique.*Br J Dermatol.* 2000 Feb;142(2):338-9.

[211] Thomas M, Pim D, Banks L.The role of the E6-p53 interaction in the molecular pathogenesis of HPV. *Oncogene.* 1999 Dec 13;18(53):7690-700.

[212] Tilli CM, Stavast-Kooy AJ, Vuerstaek JD et al. The garlic-derived organosulfur component ajoene decreases basal cell carcinoma tumor size by inducing apoptosis. *Arch Dermatol Res.* 2003 Jul;295(3):117-23.

[213] Tokunaga N, Murakami T, Endo Y et al. Human monocyte-derived dendritic cells pulsed with wild-type p53 protein efficiently induce CTLs against p53 overexpressing human cancer cells. *Clin Cancer Res.* 2005 Feb 1;11(3):1312-8

[214] Unger T, Juven-Gershon T, Moallem E et al. Critical role for Ser20 of human p53 in the negative regulation of p53 by Mdm2. *EMBO J.* 1999 Apr 1;18(7):1805-14.

[215] van der Riet P, Nawroz H, Hruban RH et al. Frequent loss of chromosome 9p21-22 early in head and neck cancer progression.*Cancer Res.* 1994 Mar 1;54(5):1156-8.

[216] Vierboom MP, Nijman HW, Offringa et al. Tumor eradication by wild-type p53-specific cytotoxic T lymphocytes. *J Exp Med.* 1997 Aug 29;186(5):695-704.

[217] Vulliamy T, Marrone A, Goldman F et al .The RNA component of telomerase is mutated in autosomal dominant dyskeratosis congenita. *Nature.* 2001 Sep 27;413(6854):432-5.

[218] Wang LL, Levy ML, Lewis RA .Clinical manifestations in a cohort of 41 Rothmund-Thomson syndrome patients. *Am J Med Genet.* 2001 Jul 2;102(1):11- 7.

[219] Wang TY, Chen BF, Yang YC et al Histologic and immunophenotypic classification of cervical carcinomas by expression of the p53 homologue p63: a study of 250 cases. *Hum Pathol.* 2001 May;32(5):479-86.

[220] Weimar VM, Ceilley RI, Goeken JACell-mediated immunity in patients with basal and squamous cell skin cancer. *J Am Acad Dermatol.* 1980 Feb;2(2):143-7.

[221] Weinstock MA, Coulter S, Bates J et al. Human papillomavirus and widespread cutaneous carcinoma after PUVA photochemotherapy. *Arch Dermatol.* 1995 Jun;131(6):701-4.

[222] Wicking C, Smyth I, Bale A The hedgehog signalling pathway in tumorigenesis and development. *Oncogene.* 1999 Dec 20;18(55):7844-51.

[223] Wikonkal N M, Brash D E. Ultraviolet radiation induced signature mutations in photocarcinogenesis.*J Investig Dermatol Symp Proc.* 1999 Sep;4(1):6-10.

[224] Xie J, Murone M, Luoh SM et al Activating Smoothened mutations in sporadic basal-cell carcinoma *Nature.* 1998 Jan 1;391(6662):90-2.

[225] Yarosh DB, Pena AV, Nay SL et al. Calcineurin inhibitors decrease DNA repair and apoptosis in human keratinocytes following ultraviolet B irradiation. *J Invest Dermatol.* 2005 Nov;125(5):1020-5.

[226] Yengi L, Inskip A, Gilford J et alPolymorphism at the glutathione S-transferase locus GSTM3: interactions with cytochrome P450 and glutathione S-transferase genotypes as risk factors for multiple cutaneous basal cell carcinoma. *Cancer Res.* 1996 May 1;56(9):1974-7

[227] Yu CE, Oshima J, Fu YH, et al Positional cloning of the Werner's syndrome gene. *Science.* 1996 Apr 12;272(5259):258-62.

[228] Ziegler A, Leffell D J, Kunala S et al. Mutation hotspots due to sunlight in the p53 gene of nonmelanoma skin cancers. *Proc Natl Acad Sci U S A.* 1993 May1;90(9):4216-20.

[229] Ziegler A, Jonason AS, Leffell DJ et al. Sunburn and p53 in the onset of skin cancer. *Nature.* 1994 Dec 22-29; 372(6508):773-6.